ALEXANDER TECHNIQUE

MIKE RUSSELL

Published in 2002 by Caxton Editions
20 Bloomsbury Street
London WC1B 3JH
a member of the Caxton Publishing Group

© 2002 Caxton Publishing Group

Designed and produced for Caxton Editions
by Open Door Limited
Rutland, United Kingdom

Editing: Mary Morton
Typesetting: Jane Booth
DIGITAL IMAGERY © copyright 2002 PhotoDisc Inc.

Title: Alexander Technique
ISBN: 1 84067 302 8

IMPORTANT NOTICE
This book is not intended to be a substitute for medical
advice or treatment. Any person with a condition requiring
medical attention should consult a qualified medical
practitioner or therapist.

ALEXANDER TECHNIQUE

MIKE RUSSELL

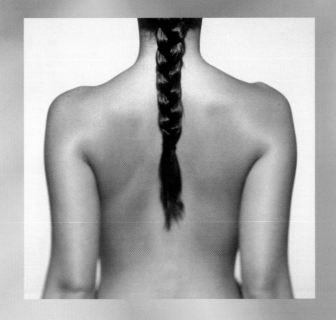

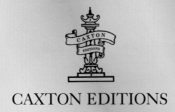

CAXTON EDITIONS

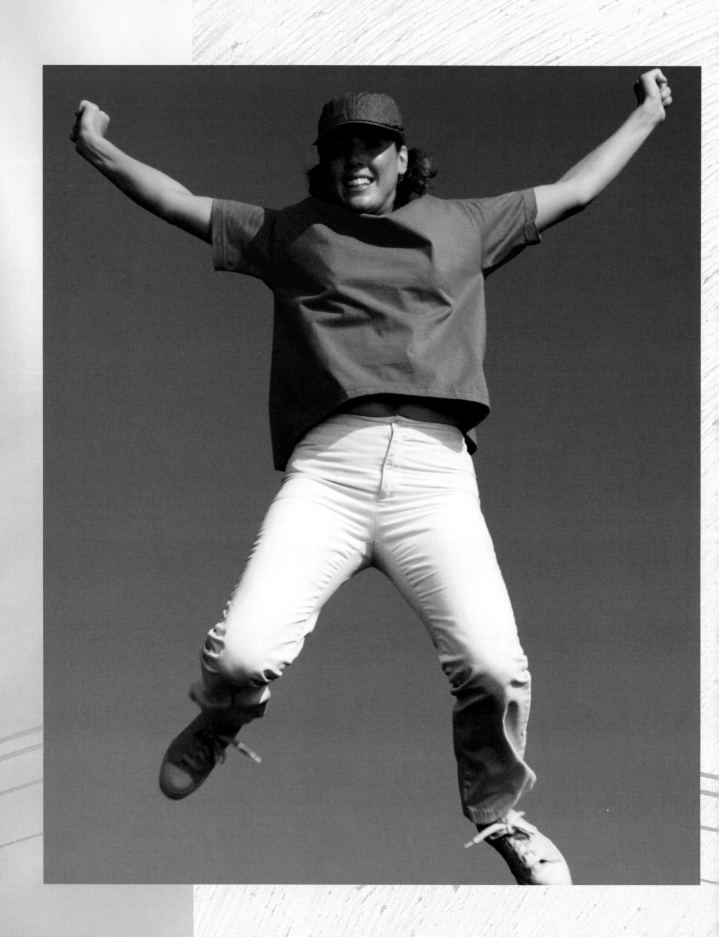

CONTENTS

INTRODUCTION   6

WHERE IT ALL STARTED   10

ALEXANDER TECHNIQUE PRINCIPLES   14

PRIMARY CONTROL   16

TAKE A BREAK: 1   47

A DAY WITH THE ALEXANDER TECHNIQUE – INDOORS   50

TAKE A BREAK: 2   61

A DAY WITH THE ALEXANDER TECHNIQUE – OUT AND ABOUT   64

TAKE A BREAK: 3   74

A DAY WITH THE ALEXANDER TECHNIQUE – BACK INDOORS   76

TAKE A BREAK: 4   86

CONCLUSIONS AND SUMMARY   88

USEFUL ADDRESSES   92

FURTHER READING   93

INDEX   94

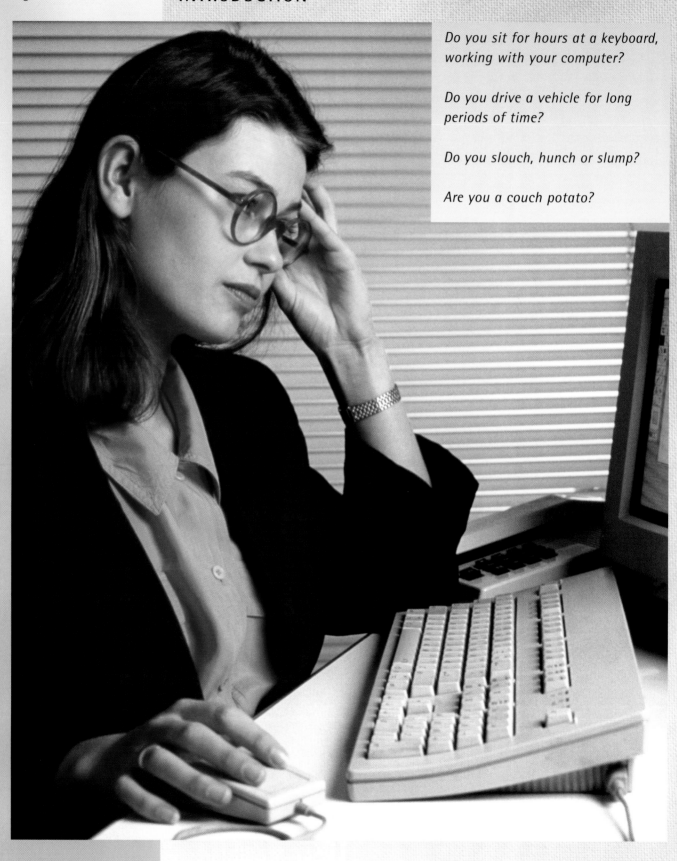

Do you sit for hours at a keyboard, working with your computer?

Do you drive a vehicle for long periods of time?

Do you slouch, hunch or slump?

Are you a couch potato?

If the answer to any of these questions is 'yes', then you probably suffer from aches and pains. Why? Because all of the above situations are linked to bad posture. Unless you are conscious of how you sit, working at a keyboard can cause back problems and repetitive strain injury (RSI) can occur. Driving for long spells of time is one of the major causes of backache known to modern man – and woman. Slouching is bad for your overall posture, especially your spine and your breathing. Couch potatoes allow their spines to curve to such an extent that they are unable to stand up straight or fill their lungs correctly.

Our bodies are built to be dynamic and, except when asleep, to keep moving. If we are static for any length of time, we try to ease the tension by slumping. This is true whether we are standing or sitting. Allowing the body to sag like this has a detrimental effect on both the muscles and joints and is harmful to the spine. And this is where the pain comes in.

Poor posture can also have other bad effects on our bodies and the way that they function. This can set off a chain of events that can lead to all-round poor health. For example, sitting in a slumped position during or after a meal can cause digestive problems, due to the gut being compressed and thus closed to the passage of food. As we all know, an upset stomach can lead to irritability and this in turn can cause emotional problems – and so the list goes on.

Look at any baby or young child and you will notice how they sit and stand straight as nature intended. Why? Because they are always on the move and never retain a static position for more than a minute. We say that our children are restless and fidgety, but they are naturally and unconsciously flexing their muscles and moving their joints.

Far left: slouching is bad for your overall posture, especially your spine and your breathing.

Below: are you a couch potato?

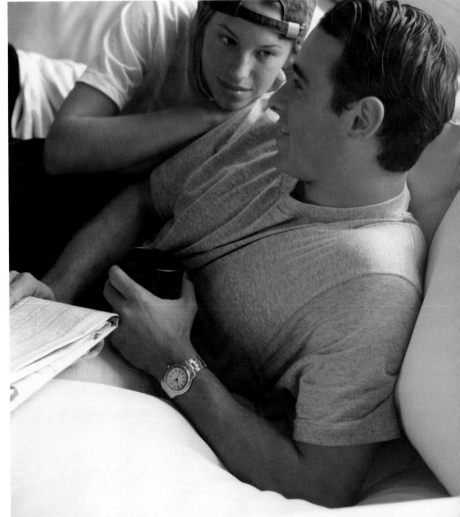

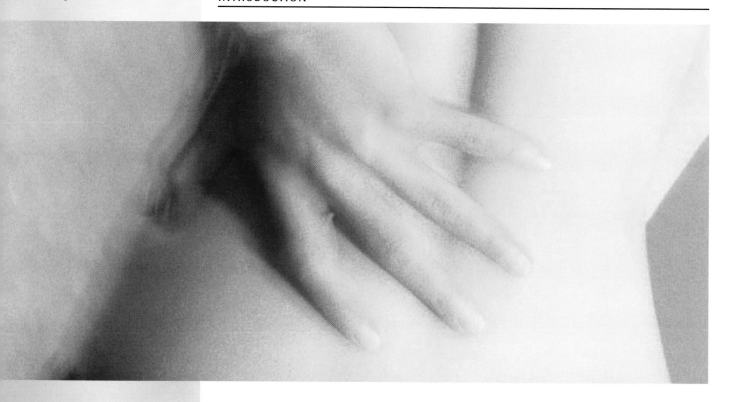

Above: nearly half the population of this country suffers from some form of back trouble.

It is estimated that nearly half the population of this country suffers from some form of back trouble, at considerable cost to the NHS. More working days are lost through back pain than any other complaint. Most of these problems would be eliminated if we could return to the posture that our bodies were intended to have – that adopted by babies and young children.

Not all back problems are caused by sitting or standing incorrectly. Much of the strain can be caused by not using our backs properly when we go about our everyday tasks. Lifting heavy objects, gardening, even rising from a chair are all notorious for causing trouble. But there are many more everyday activities that can put our bodies in jeopardy without us realising it.

Cleaning windows, pushing a vacuum cleaner, getting out of the bath, playing a musical instrument, writing, carrying a shopping bag and even turning taps on and off can all cause strain. As a result we suffer from RSI, as already mentioned, tenosynovitis, regional pain syndrome, frozen shoulder, writers' cramp, tennis elbow – etc.

As the author, Goldenthwaite, said in *Body Mechanics*: 'An individual is in the best health only when the body is so used that there is no strain on any of its parts. This means that when standing the body is held fully erect, with no strain on the joints, bones, ligaments, muscles or any other structures. There should be adequate room for all the viscera, so that their function can be performed normally.'

To do this we need to realise – and remember – that our minds and bodies must work together, in complete harmony. We need some system, a method by which we can re-train our bodies to follow the above advice in a natural manner.

This is the mind-body connection that is at the root of the Alexander Technique.

Here is a method, devised by one man, F M Alexander, that shows us how to move our bodies in the way that they were meant to move, as well as rest and relax them in the way that nature intended. If we follow his technique, we will get rid of our bad postural habits because we will be taking conscious control of our bodies.

There are other benefits, too, of using the Alexander Technique that may not be immediately obvious, such as improvement for those suffering from high blood pressure, bad sleep patterns, breathing problems, depression and an inability to cope with life in general.

Below: we get rid of our bad postural habits by taking conscious control of our bodies.

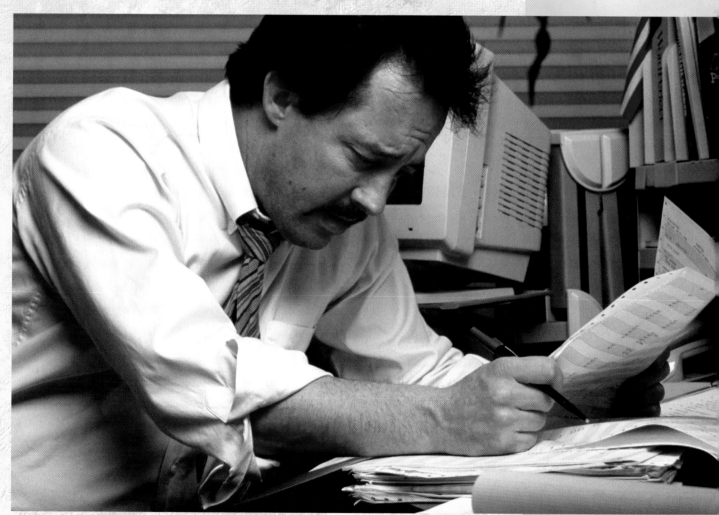

WHERE IT ALL STARTED

In the late nineteenth century. Frederick Matthias Alexander, an Australian actor from whom the technique takes its name, kept losing his voice. He found that this only happened when he was on stage, delivering his lines. At other times he had no problem. Being an inquisitive man, he wanted to know why this should happen. Nobody could tell him. Back home he set up some mirrors so that he could watch himself, from all angles, while making his speeches.

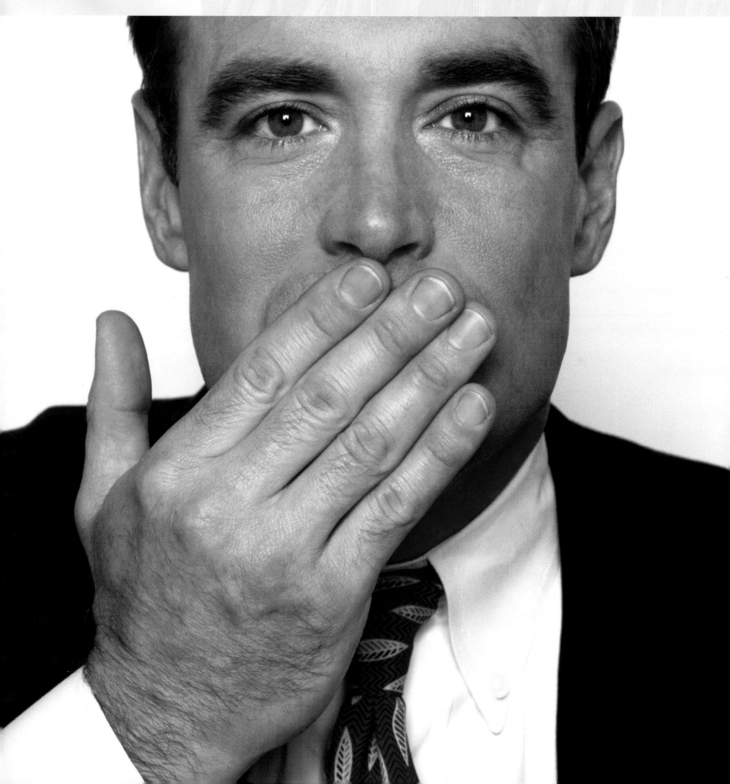

First, he spoke his lines in his normal, everyday, at-home voice. Everything looked and felt fine. What he was not prepared for was the difference that he saw in the mirrors when he adopted his stage stance and delivery. He saw that he hollowed his back, raised his chest and stiffened his neck as he retracted his head. His larynx became depressed and he was sucking air in through his mouth. Sure enough, as he continued with his delivery these stresses and strains caused him to lose his voice. He found that if he improved his posture and relaxed, he could still make his stage delivery, but his voice was no longer strained.

Alexander devoted himself to finding out how he could develop his new idea and then use it to help others.

Over the next 10 years he studied his own movements – walking, gesturing, talking, standing and sitting. What he saw led him to the conclusion that the position of his head, neck and spine was the major factor in the tensions that developed in the rest of his body.

By consciously re-aligning his body, he found that he was more relaxed, his breathing was better, and his acting and voice improved.

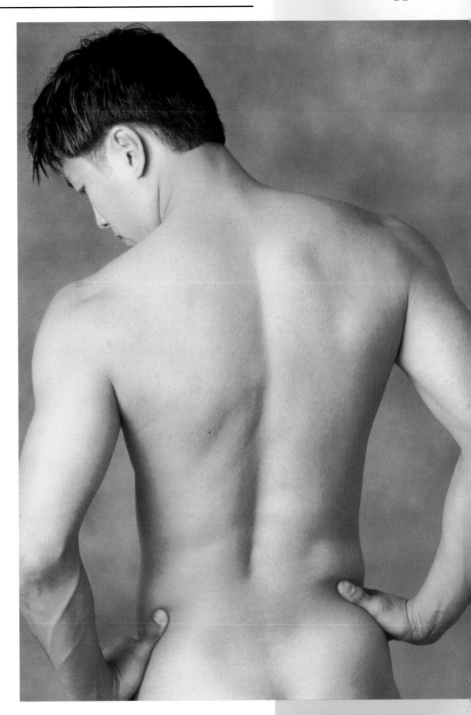

Above: the position of the head, neck and spine is a major factor in the tensions that developed in the rest of the body.

Right: Alexander first taught his technique in Australia., and then came to London where, in 1904, he opened his first school.

It was not long before other actors and speakers heard of his achievement and came to him for advice. Thus the Alexander Technique was born.

He first taught his technique in Australia, and then came to London where, in 1904, Alexander opened his first school – a training school for teachers. Wishing to spread his message further, he started to lecture and went on a successful tour of America. It should be noted here that, throughout this period, he never once experienced any trouble with his voice. He was his own best advertisement.

In 1924 he set up an infant school in London. Here children were taught to retain their innate habits of good posture, and prevented from developing those bad habits that he knew to be all too common. This school continued in England until World War II when it successfully transferred to America.

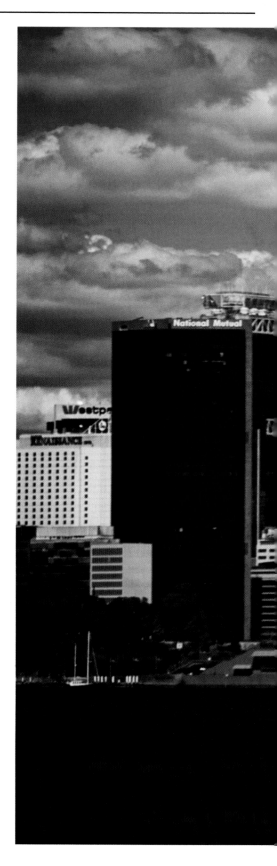

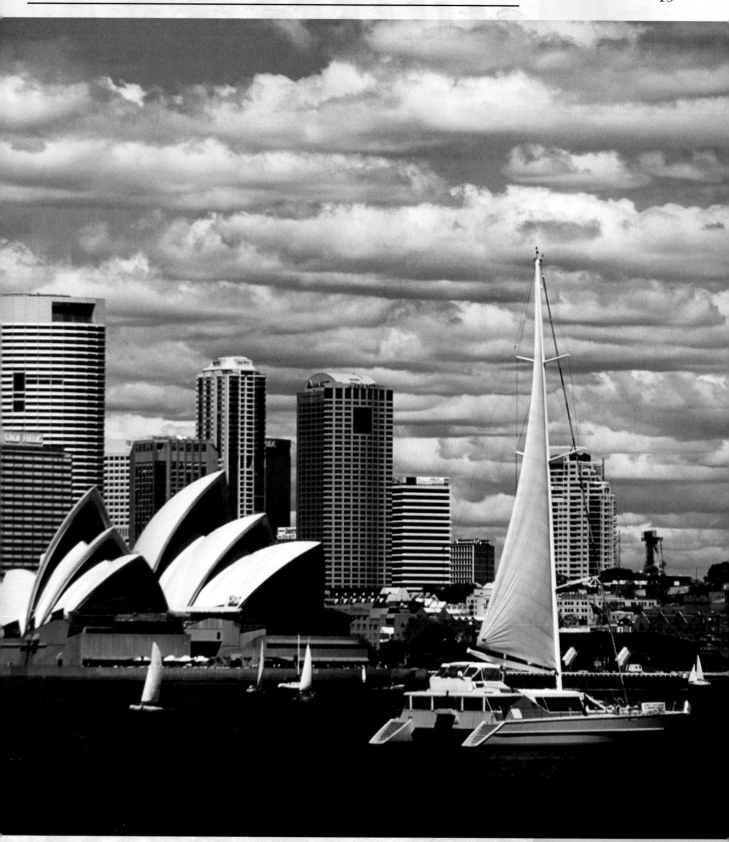

ALEXANDER TECHNIQUE PRINCIPLES

Perhaps it would be best to start by stating what the Alexander Technique is not. This will clear the way to a better understanding of what it is.

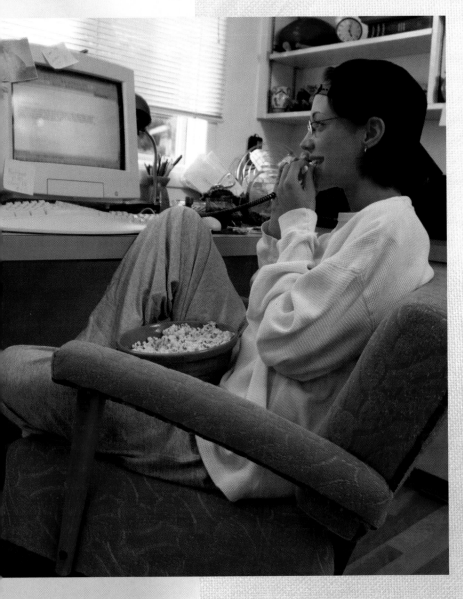

It is not an exercise that should be taken regularly to aid your posture.

It is not a routine to be undertaken as and when necessary as a temporary cure for sudden backache or loss of voice.

It is not a cure-all that can be used to remedy toothache, for instance.

It is not a religion, faith or belief.

The Alexander Technique is, as the name correctly indicates, a technique – a system or method – that will help you to lose your ingrained habits of poor posture and the resultant pain and discomfort that these bring. Alexander called these bad habits 'patterns of misuse'. If we are made aware of them, then we can learn how to re-align our bodies correctly. Thus, quite simply, the Alexander Technique aims to re-educate the body through a conscious improvement in our posture.

Above: the Alexander Technique aims to re-educate the body through a conscious improvement in our posture.

These necessary adjustments are easy to learn. They can be taught, as Alexander did, to children. First you have to learn exactly what it is that you are doing wrong, and then how to correct it. The difficult part, as we all know, is getting rid of bad habits and establishing good ones. But, with practice, it will become second nature to you.

The technique also takes into account the belief that the mind and the body are so closely linked that whatever is done to one will have an effect on the other. Alexander noted that the strain of everyday life can bring about poor posture and muscle tension. This in turn can produce a change in our physical or mental condition.

Many of your body functions, such as digestion, breathing and circulation, will be improved by using the Alexander Technique, as will your mental outlook and general feeling of well-being. If you practise the Alexander Technique, you will find that you are mentally and physically sharper than previously, but paradoxically you will also feel more relaxed. This natural state has been likened to that of an animal poised, ready for fight or flight.

One big advantage of the technique is that it can be used at any time, any place – even in a group of people without your companions being aware that you are doing anything. If asked, they may say that you look more vivacious and alert than usual, but that is all. The technique can be used when you are sitting, standing, or moving about. Moreover, once it becomes part of your life, you will find that you use it all of the time, wherever you are and whatever you are doing.

Below: the technique can be used when you are sitting, standing, or moving about.

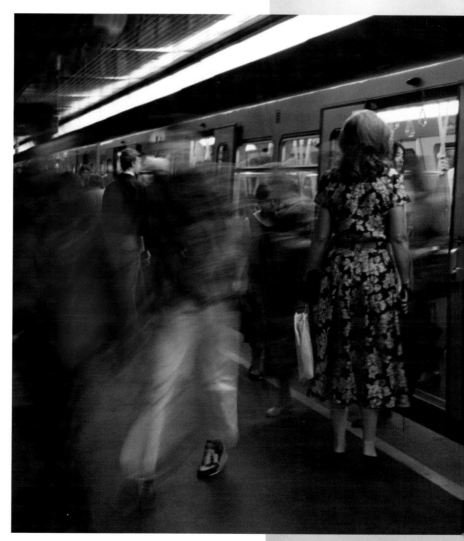

PRIMARY CONTROL

COMMON MOVEMENTS

Below: Alexander's first concept was that the head, the neck and the back should be aligned correctly.

Alexander's first concept was that the head, the neck and the back should be aligned correctly. This was later confirmed by the noted anthropologist Raymond Dart, who said, 'It is a basic biological fact that the position of the head to the neck is of primary importance in human posture and movement'.

Notice, if you have not already done so on television, how women from East Africa carry their loads. They carry their shopping, as well as their water supplies, balanced on their heads with no added support. These heavy loads are often carried over what can be very rough terrain. They perform these tasks with perfect posture and balance and also with very little fatigue. This is because they have been taught as young girls to align their heads, necks and backs so that they can carry out these tasks without consequent back problems.

Alexander called this relationship between the head, neck and back, 'primary control'. And it is with this that we will begin.

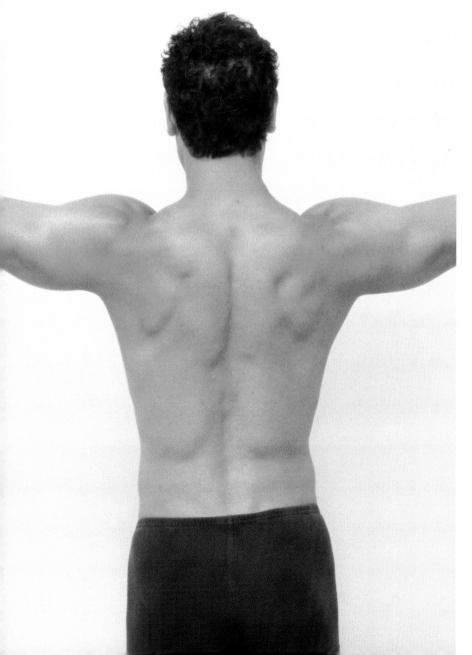

LYING DOWN

It may seem odd to be told how to lie down, but that is what this first lesson is all about. Don't feel strange that you are being asked to lie down during the day. As you will see, it is quite different from lying down in bed.

For a start you will only be lying down for 15–20 minutes. During this time you will keep your eyes open, and may not be sufficiently comfortable to fall asleep. Finally, you will be consciously thinking about what is happening to your body.

1. Find a comfortably warm, draught-free floor-space where you can lie down. Choose somewhere carpeted if possible and avoid a cold or damp floor such as tile or concrete. Before you lie down, get four or five books, each about half an inch (12 mm) thick. These are not to read, but to support your head.

Make sure before you settle down that you are not going to be disturbed for the next 20 minutes. Disconnect the door bell and the phone and put the cat out.

2. Wear some loose, comfortable clothes – a tracksuit is ideal – and remove your shoes and socks, unless it is very cold.

3. Sit down on the floor and then roll back so that your head is supported by the books. A little experimentation is needed here to find the height of head-rest to suit you. Try first with about 2 inches (50mm) of books. The aim is to support your head so that it is comfortable and feels free. Insufficient height will reduce the natural curve of the neck, while too many books will push your head forward and restrict your breathing.

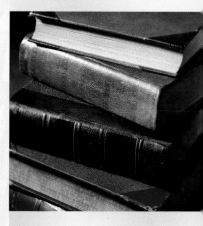

Above: before you lie down, get four or five books, each about half an inch (12 mm) thick; use fewer books if they are thicker.

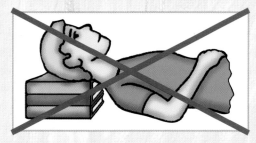

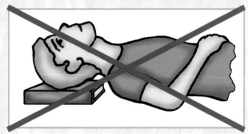

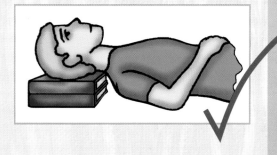

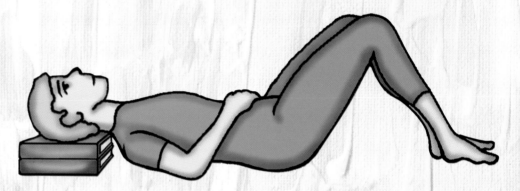

Far right: make sure that your back is as flat to the floor as is consistent with the natural arching of the back.

4. Hold your chin up, look at the ceiling, thus preventing your head from rolling to one side and keeping your airways open.

5. Moving one leg at a time, draw your feet up towards your body by bending your knees up to the ceiling. Keep your feet flat on the floor. Just bring your knees up until you are in a comfortable, relaxed position, with your feet slightly wider apart than your shoulders or the width of your pelvis. They should be about 18 inches (45cm) apart.

6. Make sure that your back is as flat to the floor as is consistent with the natural arching of the back. If it is not, adjust your position by moving your bottom. This usually means that you will need to increase the distance between your bottom and your shoulders, straightening your back a little while retaining the natural hollowness there.

7. Your hands should now be placed just above your waist, on the lower ribs, keeping your elbows on the floor, the fingertips of one hand just touching those of the other. Feel your body settle into the floor and, as you do so, check that your chest is relaxed by letting out a large sigh.

8. If you have taken up this position correctly, you will find that your body is supported at nine points – your head, your two shoulders, your two elbows, your hips and your two feet. In this semi-supine position your spine is well supported and your whole body is free from those tensions that so often cause bad posture. Your rib cage will be relaxed and open, which reduces the pressure on your lungs and is also good for your diaphragm. This position removes all restrictions from your breathing and provides the necessary room for your internal organs to take up their natural positions.

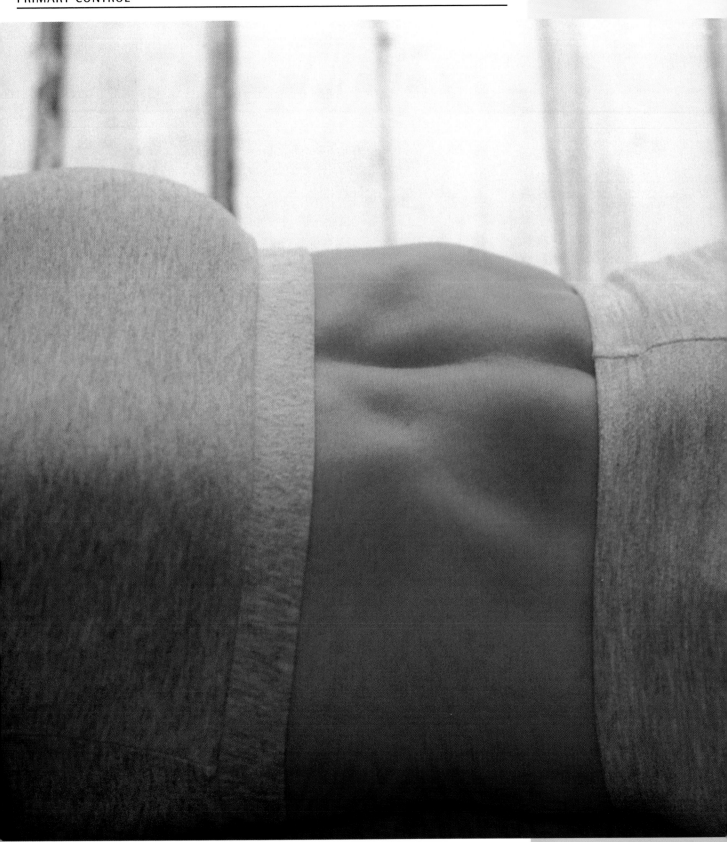

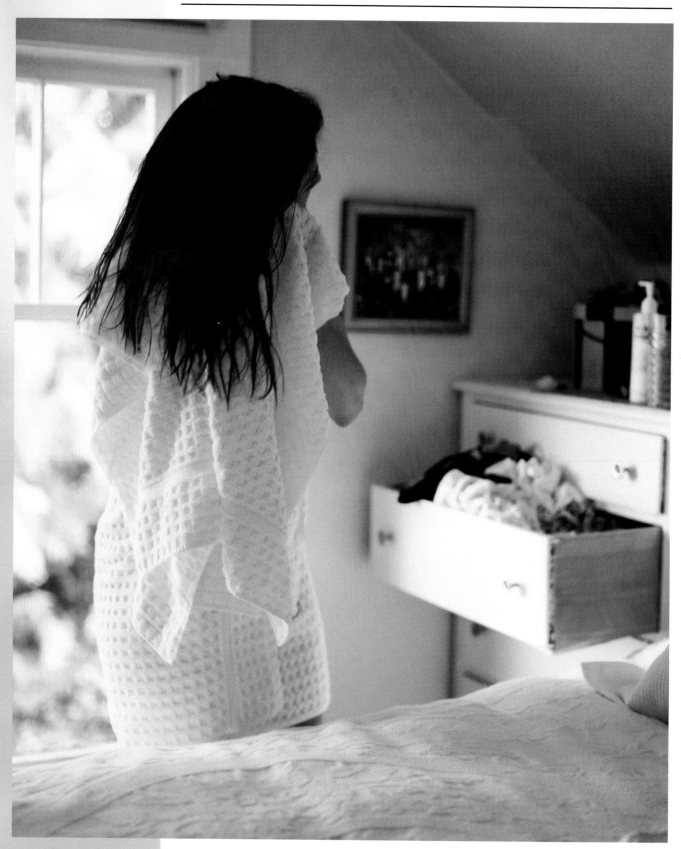

9. If your back has been troubling
you, you may find it difficult to relax
at the outset. This is most often
evident in a tension that won't allow
you to sink into the floor, as you
should. If this occurs, you will notice
that there is a large hollow beneath
your lower back. Don't worry about
this. Just relax as much as possible for
five minutes. Then, place your hands
under your pelvis and try to move
your lower back further away from
the top of your spine. Place a little
tension in your knees and ankles to
help move your pelvis. Repeat this
after a further five minutes. This will
gently stretch your spine as the
tension is released. You may be
surprised at how your spine has
relaxed and, as a result, stretched.
This happens because the weight of
your head and shoulders has been
taken off your spine, and the stress is
removed from your shoulders.

It is a fact that when we get out of
bed in the morning we are taller than
we were when we went to bed the
previous night. This is because our
spines actually lengthen as the
intervertebral discs become
decompressed as a result of not
bearing the weight of our bodies and
heads.

*Far left: when we get
out of bed in the
morning we are taller
than we were when we
went to bed.*

*Below: you may be
surprised at how your
spine has relaxed and,
as a result, stretched.*

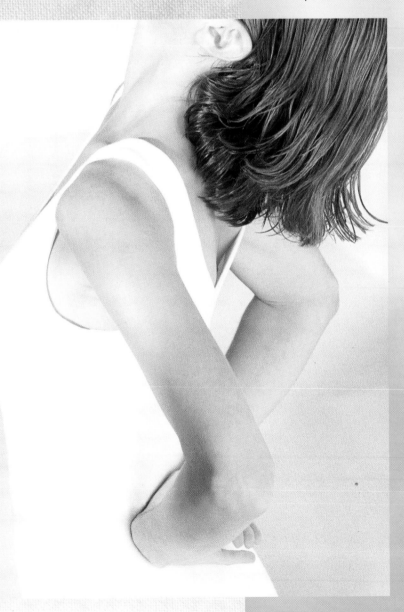

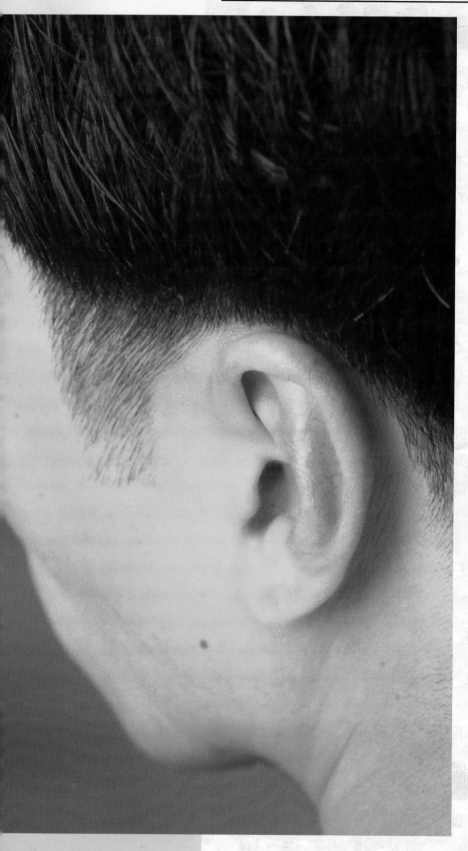

10. As you lay there, with your body relaxed, it is time to start thinking. We all think, all the time that we are awake. This act of thinking uses the brain and the brain uses oxygen. The more you think, the more oxygen you need; the more oxygen you need, the deeper you will have to breathe. Think about this. Become aware of your thoughts. Even when you are not consciously thinking of anything your senses are still alert. Take particular note of them now.

11. Be aware of your hands on your ribs, rising and falling rhythmically. Feel the texture of the material beneath them. Feel the books beneath your head and the carpet under your elbows.

12. Listen to what sounds there are. What can you hear? If nothing else, you should be able to hear your heart beating.

13. Feel the air moving through your nostrils. Don't force it, or try to speed it up – just be aware of what is happening. Think about your breath going in, and out, in and out. At the same time notice any smell that there may be.

14. Remember to keep your eyes open. Observe the ceiling. Are there odd patterns there that you had not noticed before? As you become more relaxed, you may find that you do tend to drop off to sleep. If this happens, take two or three sharp intakes of breath to fill your lungs to capacity before exhaling as much as possible and completely emptying them. Do this three or four times and you will find that you are wide awake again.

Far left: listen to what sounds there are. What can you hear?

Below: remember to keep your eyes open. Observe the ceiling.

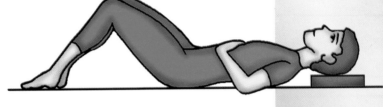

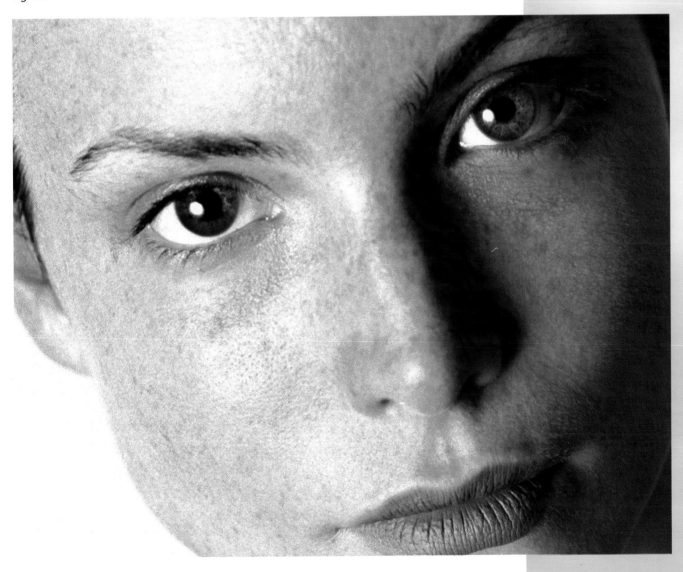

15. Next, imagine that you are sinking into the floor.
Think about this.

Feel your head sinking through the books. Think about this.

Feel your shoulders sinking into the floor. Think about this.

Feel your hips sinking into the floor. Think about this.

Feel your elbows sinking into the floor. Think about this.

Feel your feet sinking into the floor. Think about this.

Feel your spine lengthening. Think about this.

Feel your joints loosening as they relax. Think about this.

16. When you have lain in the semi-supine position for 15–20 minutes, bring your thoughts back to your breath. You will be surprised at how much it has altered. It will be more rhythmic, shallower and slower that when you first lay down. You have relaxed.

Once you are sure of the correct thickness of books to support your head, buy a block of polystyrene foam, or some similar material that gives you the support, without being quite so hard. This is not a course in masochism – you should be as comfortable and relaxed as possible.

Six steps to lying down:

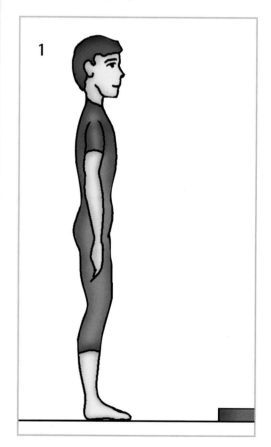

1

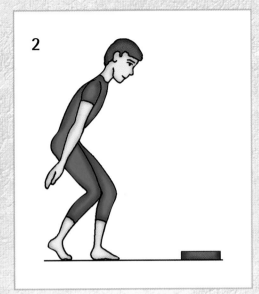

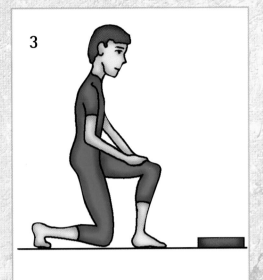

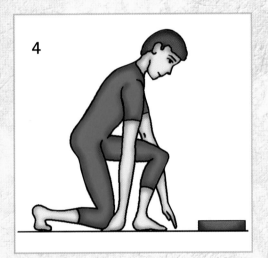

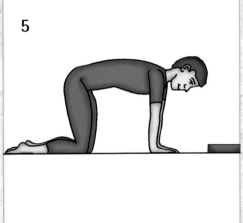

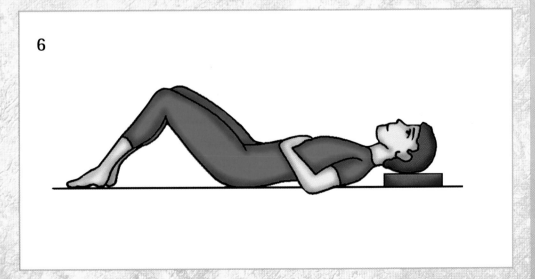

START POSITION

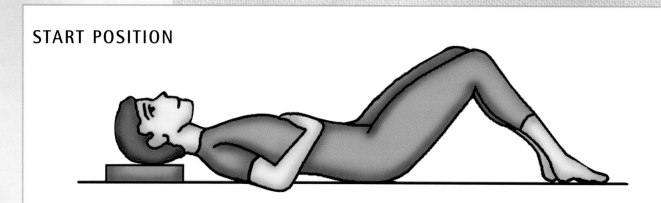

3

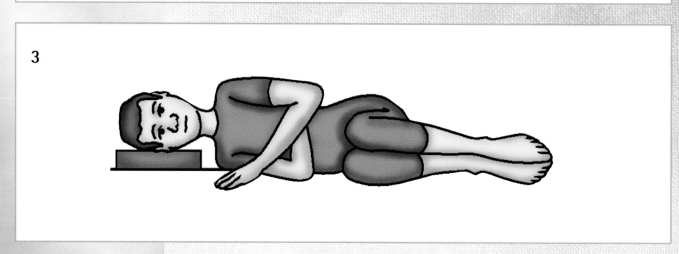

5

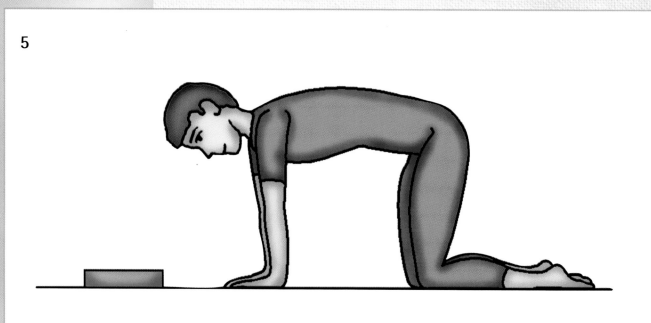

GETTING UP

Now we come to the final part of lying down – and that is getting up. If you thought it odd that you were told how to lie down, you may think it completely off-the-wall to be told how to get up. Nevertheless there is only one correct way to do this. If you don't get up correctly, there is a chance that you will undo all the good gained by lying down.

It is important that you take your time when getting up. If you were able to allow sufficient time for lying down, there should be no reason for you now to jump up and dash off. Don't be tempted to rush the process at any point.

1. Raise one arm with your hand pointing up to the ceiling, breathing in as you do so.

2. Move that arm across your body, letting it slowly fall.

3. As it comes down, roll over on to that side.

4. Stop at this point while you exhale. Keep your body relaxed.

5. Continue rolling over until you are face down, on all fours, in a crawling position.

6. Hold this position while you take another breath.

7. Slowly rock backwards and forwards until you can sit back on your heels.

Far left: if you don't get up correctly, there is a chance that you will undo all the good gained by lying down.

Below: it is important that you take your time when getting up

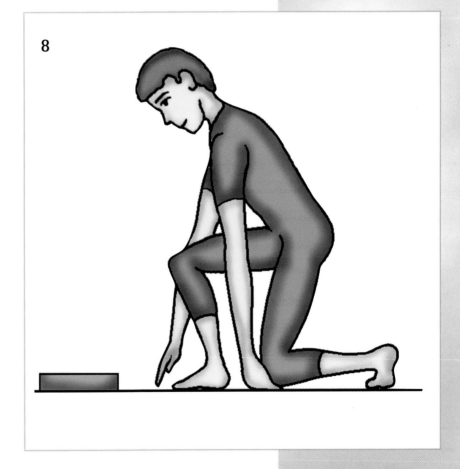

8

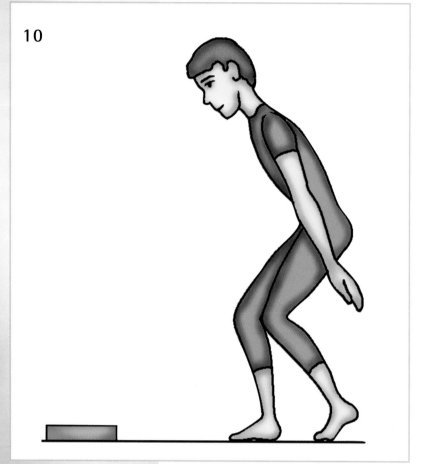

10

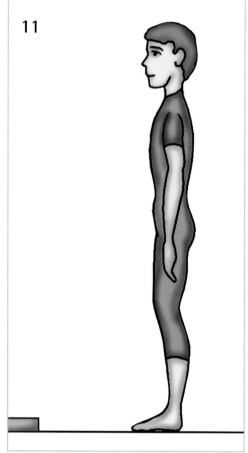

11

Far right: if at any time you feel tensed up, for whatever reason, lie down again and actively relax.

8. From this position push yourself up and bring one leg forward so that your foot is flat on the ground and you are kneeling on the other leg.

9. Rest again and check your breathing and that your body is still relaxed.

10. Keeping your body upright, push up on the forward leg and bring your other leg alongside to regain a full standing position.

11. Stand for a moment to take another breath before moving off.

This business of standing up sounds much more complicated than it is. When you attempt it, you will find that it is an easy and natural way to stand.

If at any time you feel tensed up, for whatever reason, lie down again and actively relax. Remain there until you are sure that when you get up, you can still remain loose, both mentally and physically.

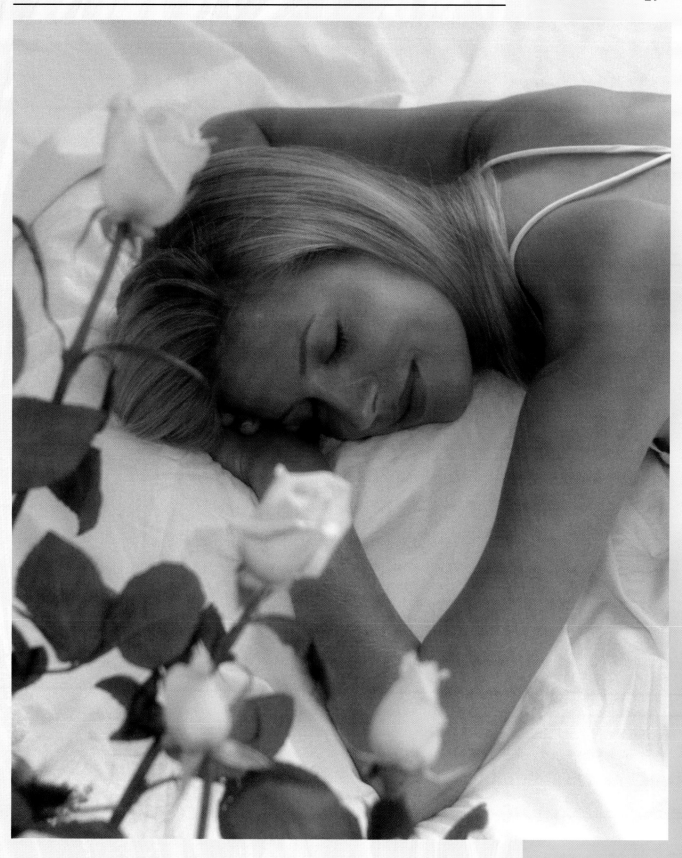

STANDING

To be able to stand correctly, relaxed and without any tension, is something that we all forget almost as soon as we leave infant school. If you can learn to stand properly, you will find that it is far less tiring, your breathing is easier and you will lose mental as well as physical tension.

Below: watch anyone standing at a bus stop and you will see common bad habits which have developed in us all when we have to stand anywhere for any length of time.

Through the years we gradually take on the habit of standing for any length of time by bracing ourselves. Then, becoming tired of this, we slump down. Eventually we need to support our bodies on the nearest stable object to prevent ourselves from falling over.

Watch anyone standing at a bus stop and you will see what I mean. First they take their weight on one foot and brace that leg, leaning on one hip with the back twisted. Then they move their weight to the other foot and do the same again. Next they slump down, flat-footed on both feet, usually leaning back, stomach protruding and twisting their spine at the same time. Finally they prop their body up against the bus shelter or nearest wall. The longer they stand, the more tense and tired they become.

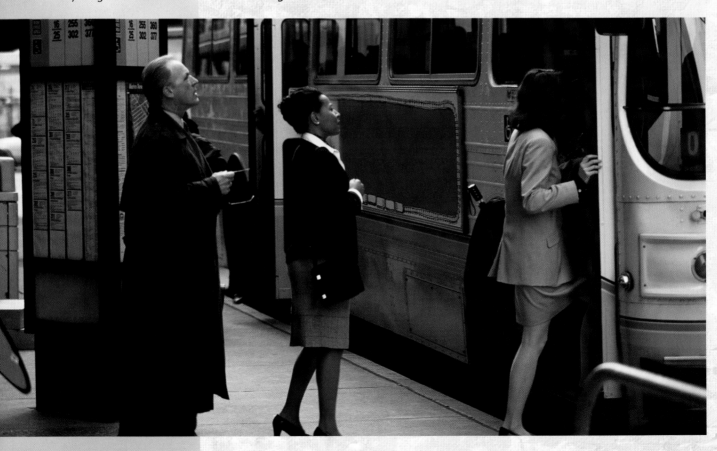

There is no need for this. It is quite possible to stand for long periods, quite comfortably and relaxed, if you stand correctly. Alexander gave his pupils – as he called all those who came under his tuition – a set of instructions that he called 'conscious projections'. These were to be memorised and repeated, so that they became rather like a mantra, their message becoming embedded at the sub-conscious level. You will find that I repeat them at regular intervals throughout this book.

Recite them frequently until you have learned them thoroughly:

Let the neck be free.

Let the head go forwards and up.

Allow the back to lengthen and widen.

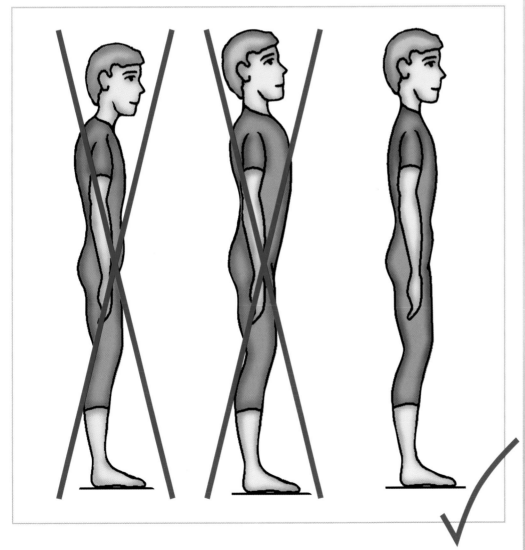

Left: standing positions; a slouched position (left) over extended (centre) and the correct position – it is quite possible to stand for long periods, quite comfortably and relaxed, if you stand correctly.

3

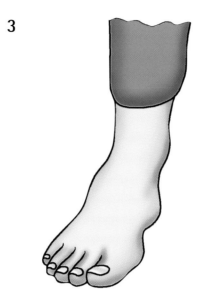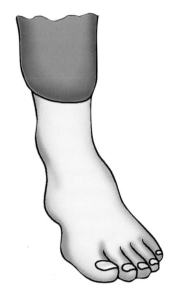

Above: place your feet with your weight evenly distributed between them.

The exercise of these projections was known as 'primary control'. All those who attempt the Alexander Technique are advised to practise this control and strive to make it second nature.

With these three points in mind:

1. Remove any footwear.

2. Shake each arm in turn to loosen up the muscles and then allow them to relax and hang by your sides, fingers loose.

3. Place your feet somewhat less than shoulder width apart with your weight evenly distributed between them.

4. Don't splay your feet so far that they are at right angles to one another and don't point them straight ahead. Aim for something in between.

5. Check that your feet are flat on the floor. Lean very slightly forward so that the weight on each foot is equally distributed between your heel, a point just behind your big toe and the pad behind your small toe – thus forming a tripod.

6. Become aware of your toes on the ground, helping you to maintain your balance.

7. Lean over to one side and lift one foot off the ground. Become conscious of those three points taking all your weight on the other foot and ensure that it is equally distributed between them.

8. Go back on to both feet and then lean the other way, lift the other foot and again be aware of your weight distribution.

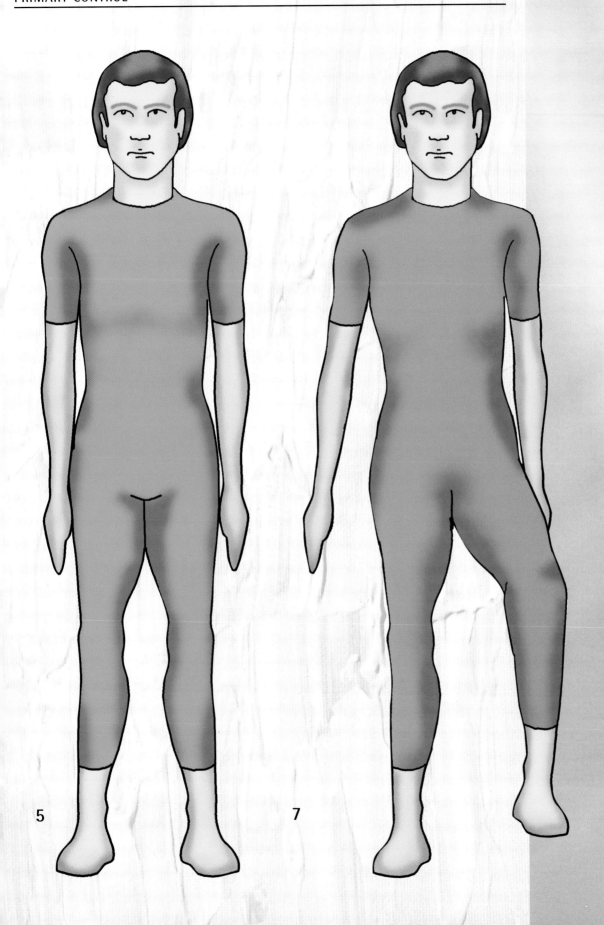

5   7

Far right: being able to walk correctly follows on quite naturally from being able to stand the way that we should.

Below: move your head in a loose circle to relax your neck. Then circle it the other way.

9. Settle back down on to both feet again, making sure that your legs are straight without your knees being locked and pressed back. If you are correctly balanced, this will not happen. If your knees are braced, lean back slightly and let your knees bend somewhat.

10. Straighten your back without stiffening it.

11. Move your head in a loose circle to relax your neck. Then circle it the other way.

12. Finish with your head facing forward and hanging comfortably before lifting it slightly as though looking out to the horizon. Your head is now 'forward and up,' the second of Alexander's conscious projections.

13. Take a breath in and lift both shoulders.

14. Move your shoulders back slightly and, as you exhale, allow them to drop, but not to fall forward.

15. You should finish with your back wider and longer than before.

You are now standing, relaxed and balanced with no tension to tire you. Stay there for a few moments until you become conscious of how comfortable it can be to stand correctly. As you stand there, bear in mind the 'conscious projections'.

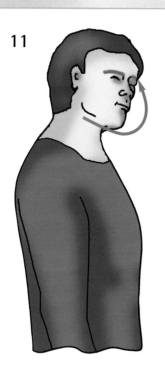
11

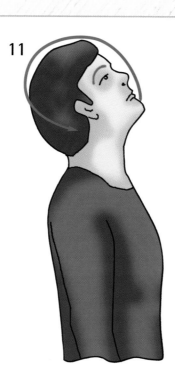
11

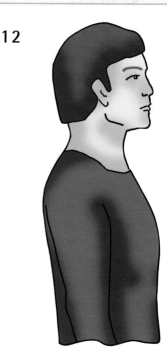
12

WALKING

Suggesting that you learn how to walk may seem rather like teaching your grandmother how to suck eggs. It is true that you will find the movements simplistic and not much related to the everyday walking you have been doing. But do practise them and gradually you will find that you build on them to achieve a natural, but improved, walk.

Being able to walk correctly follows on quite naturally from being able to stand the way that we should.

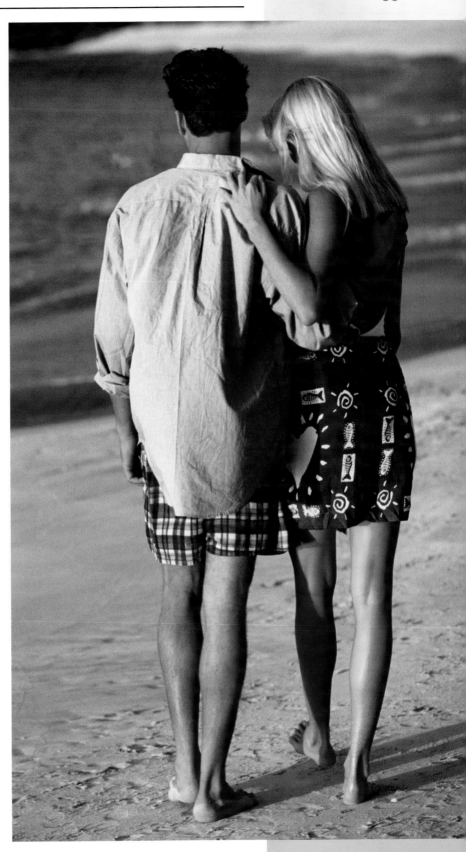

1. Stand for a moment in the position already learned.

2. As you breathe out, lift one heel, bending the knee, but keeping the ball of the foot on the ground.

3. Lower your heel as you breathe in, so that it returns to its original position.

4. Repeat this rocking motion a few times, becoming aware of the flexing of your hip, knee, ankle and foot.

5. Feel this as an easy, rhythmic motion that is done with hardly any weight on heel or toe.

6. Do the same with your other foot.

7. As you breathe out again, lift your leg so that your foot comes completely off the floor – but only just.

8. Swing your foot straight ahead so that it is just in front of the foot that is taking your weight. While doing this, keep your weight over your back foot.

9. Now allow your body to start to move by leaning forward slightly. Make sure that your back is kept straight.

10. Allow your weight to transfer to your forward foot as your rear knee bends.

Below: as you breathe out lift one heel (2), bending the knee, but keeping the ball of the foot on the ground.

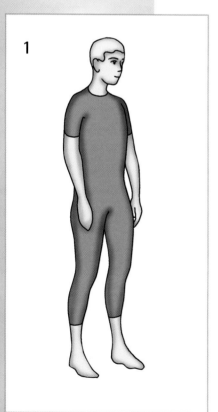

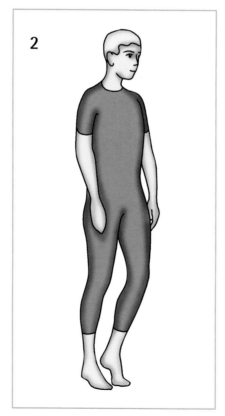

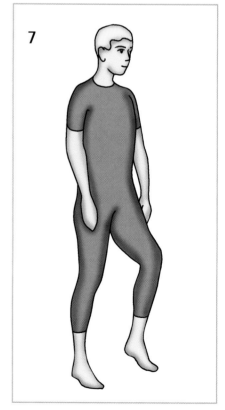

11. At the same time the rear heel should be allowed to rise as you prepare to repeat the whole operation with your other leg.

12. Keep your body and head facing forward so that your spine is not twisted. The whole movement should come from the hips down, in a natural and flowing rhythm.

13. Allow your arms to swing freely. As you pick up pace, you will find that your arms will naturally move counter to your feet – left foot and right arm forward and then right foot and left arm forward. This helps to retain your balance and rhythm. Don't force your arms forward and swing them like a soldier on parade; just let them move naturally.

If you can watch yourself in a mirror as you walk – or perhaps in shop windows – you will note that if you are moving correctly, as suggested, your body appears to float along with an almost imperceptible rise and fall. Your head should not be bobbing up and down. Watch a cat as it walks and you will see what is meant here. It appears to roll ahead as though on casters.

Once you have mastered walking steadily with good poise, you will find that this technique can be improved and reinforced by practising walking backwards. This little diversion is very good for the balance. Keep your head forward and up as you walk backwards, but make sure that there is sufficient clear space behind you before setting off.

Below: watch yourself as you walk, perhaps in shop windows.

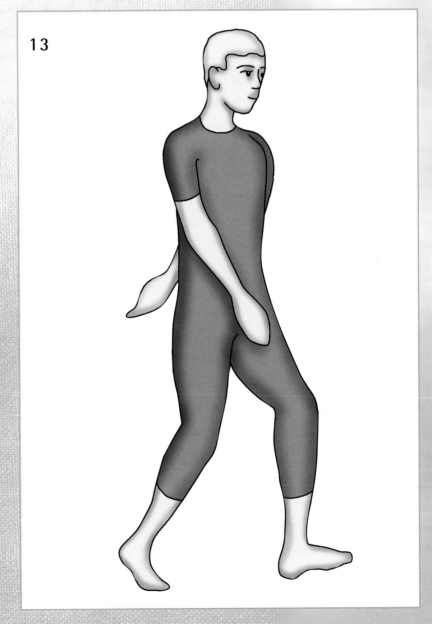

13

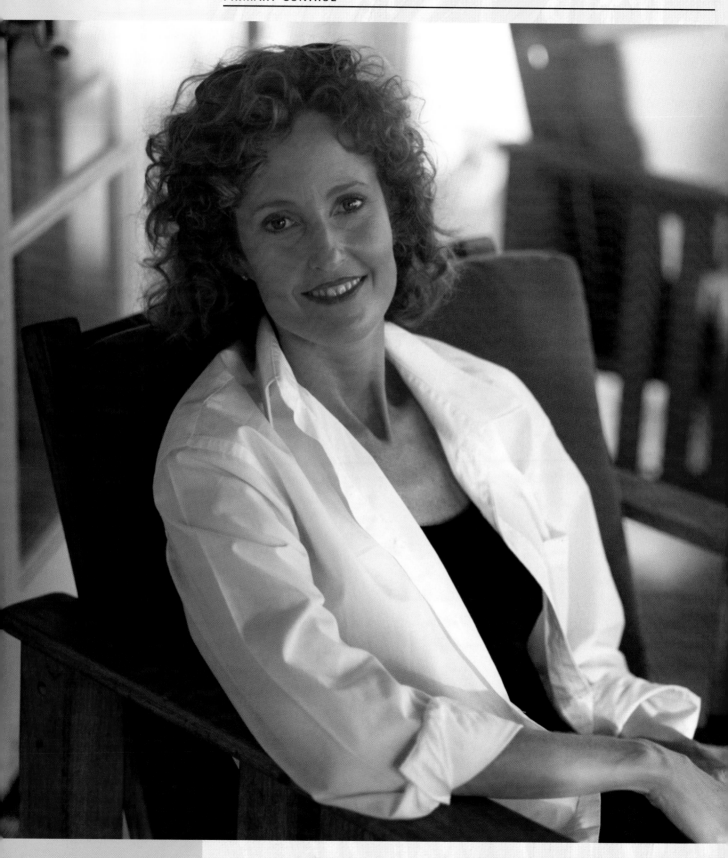

SITTING DOWN

After all that walking you will probably want to sit down. But do you sit down correctly? Probably not. This is because, although chairs were designed for us to sit on, our bodies were not designed for the chairs.

As most of us spend several hours a day sitting down, it is important that we sit correctly. Again, the procedure is easy to learn and, in this case, easily remembered.

Start by taking a straight-backed chair with a hard, level seat – a dining-chair is ideal.

Far left: do you sit down correctly?

Below: it is important that we sit correctly.

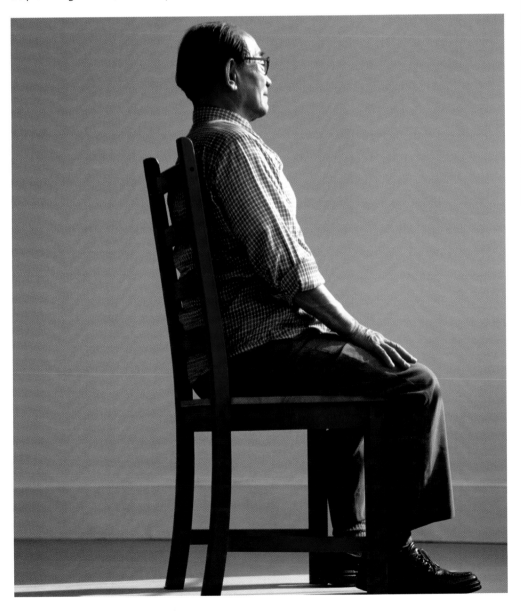

1. Stand 5 or 6 inches (12–15cm) in front of the chair, with your back to it, in the natural relaxed standing position, feet at slightly less than shoulder width apart, weight evenly distributed.

2. Make sure that your body is relaxed as you lean forward and breathe out.

3. Move your hips back by bending your knees and at the same time bend your body forward from the hips as a counterbalance.

4. Continue to keep your back straight and your head forward and up as you sink down.

5. This should bring you into a position where you are sitting in the chair, leaning slightly forward.

6. As the weight has been taken off your feet, you can now straighten up from the hips to bring your spine and head upright.

7. Place your hands on your thighs and you will be completely relaxed and comfortable.

Below: although chairs were designed for us to sit on, our bodies were not designed for the chairs.

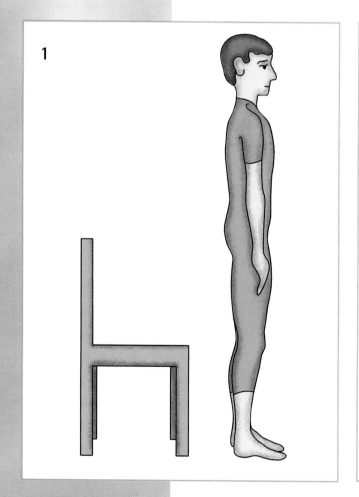

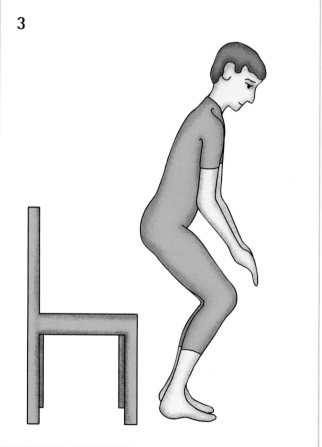

Having sat down, we now need to look at the sitting position. If you sit well back in your chair, you will feel the base of the chair-back supporting your lumber regions, as it should. Don't sit so that you are perched on the edge of the chair. If you do so and then lean back, you will have your weight on the base of the coccyx (last bone of the spinal column) instead of the two lower parts of the pelvis. This leads to back pain and consequent damage.

Below: place your hands on your thighs and you will be completely relaxed and comfortable.

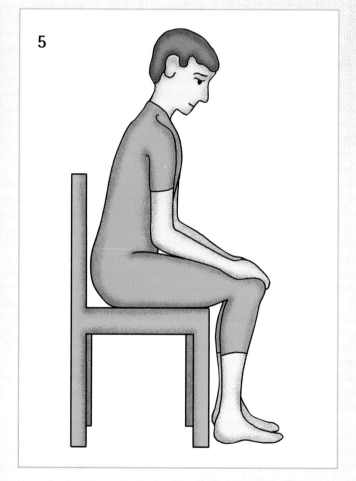

5

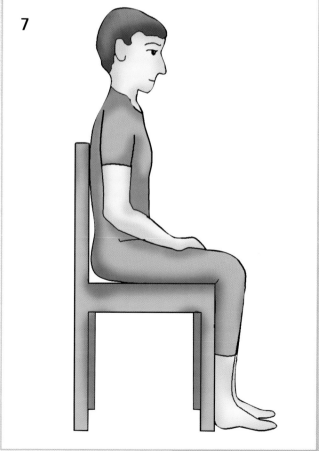

7

Below: men have the habit of crossing their legs so that one calf is resting on the other knee.

While sitting down you may move your feet to a limited extent. Most women will naturally move their feet together as they sit. But do try to avoid leaning your knees over to one side, thus twisting the hips and pelvis – a common habit if the chair is low. Similarly, men have the habit of crossing their legs so that one calf is resting on the other knee. This is bad for the blood circulation and should also be avoided. On the other hand, crossing the feet at the ankles does no harm, though it is better to keep both feet flat on the floor.

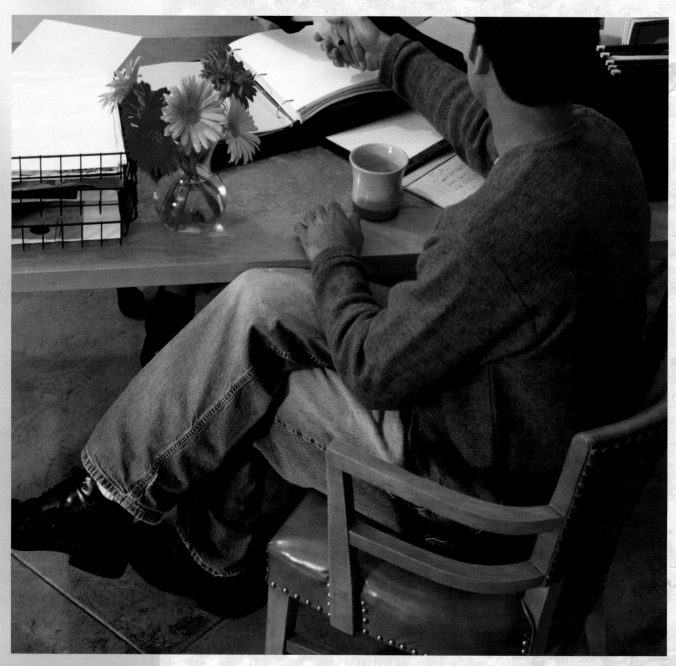

STANDING UP AGAIN

The way to get out of the chair is simple. All you have to do is reverse the method of sitting down. Lead with your head. Let it fall forward so that your body follows. In the archives there is a film of Alexander doing just this, and if the film is run backwards it is impossible to tell whether he is going through the motion of standing up or sitting down. There should be absolutely no difference between the two.

Sitting in an easy chair requires special attention. First, take a look at the chair. If it is too deep, from front to back-cushion, place some support for your lower back. When you sit down in it, beware of then allowing your body to flop, as is customary. Try to maintain a position where you remain more or less upright. This may mean sitting to one side of the chair and using the arm for some support. The main danger is in slouching so that you are sitting on the base of your spine rather than on your pelvis.

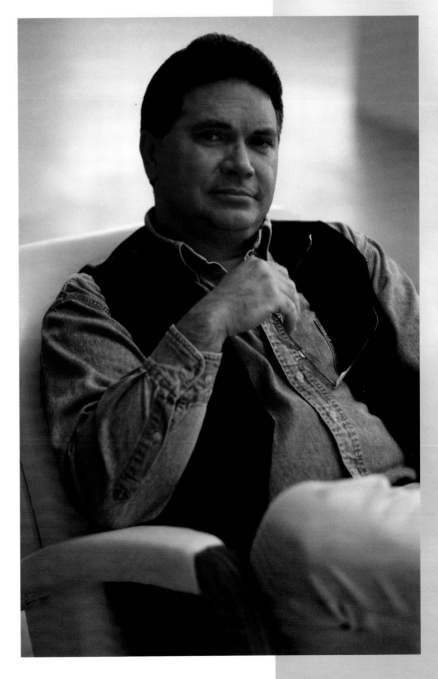

Below: sitting in an easy chair requires special attention..

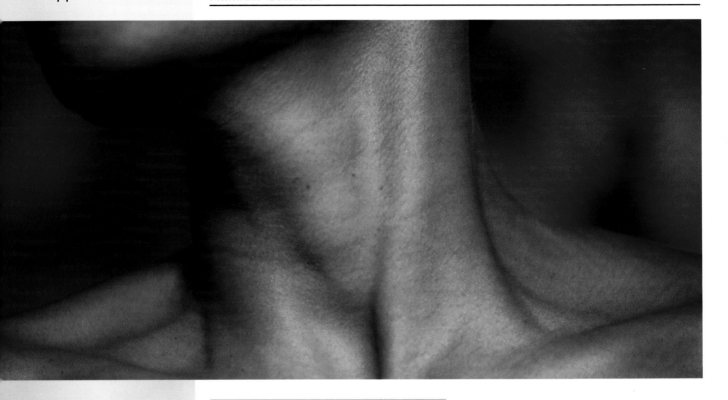

Above: tension causes our chest muscles to tighten and impede our full intake of air.

BREATHING

This last section of the fundamentals of the Alexander Technique brings us back to its origins. If you remember, it was Alexander's loss of voice that started off this whole idea. Loss of voice, he found, equated with not breathing correctly.

The trouble is that we all breathe quite naturally, taking it for granted, and it never enters our head that we could be doing it incorrectly. We do tend to tense up our muscles in the most unexpected places. It is this tension that causes our chest muscles to tighten and impede our full intake of air.

If you have practised standing, relaxed, in the Alexander way, then you are more than halfway to breathing correctly. The main points to remember are those of the 'primary control':

Let the neck be free.

Let the head go forwards and up.

Allow the back to lengthen and widen.

In this position the airways will be clear to allow the air to travel freely into your lungs. But even so it is still possible to be tensing some muscles that prevent you breathing as easily and freely as you should.

Alexander devised an exercise to ensure that all the muscles of the neck, throat and mouth are relaxed. This is called 'The whispered Ah' and is quite simple to perform.

This exercise is especially useful for those who practise public speaking, as Alexander did, and singers, too. It allows you to make a sound without any effort, remaining completely relaxed. This is the secret of sustained performance, with no fear of voice loss.

1. Stand in front of a mirror.

2. Relax and place your hands across your waist so that your fingertips touch.

3. Gently blow air out through your mouth.

4. Use the minimum amount of effort. It should be done without moving your shoulders and with very little movement of the chest. Check this in the mirror.

5. Close your mouth before breathing in through your nose. This ensures that the air is warmed, filtered and moistened – as it should be – before entering your lungs.

6. Take the air in to your lungs steadily, in a controlled manner. Avoid sniffing.

7. Let your neck relax so that your head falls gently forward.

8. Smile and relax your mouth. It helps if you can think of something funny while doing this.

9. Place your tongue on the floor of your mouth so that its tip rests against the back of your lower teeth.

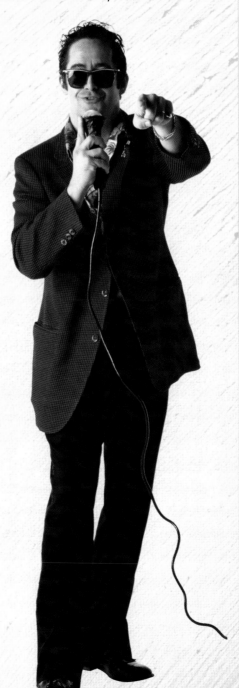

Below: people who practise public speaking and singers find 'the whispered Ah' exercise useful.

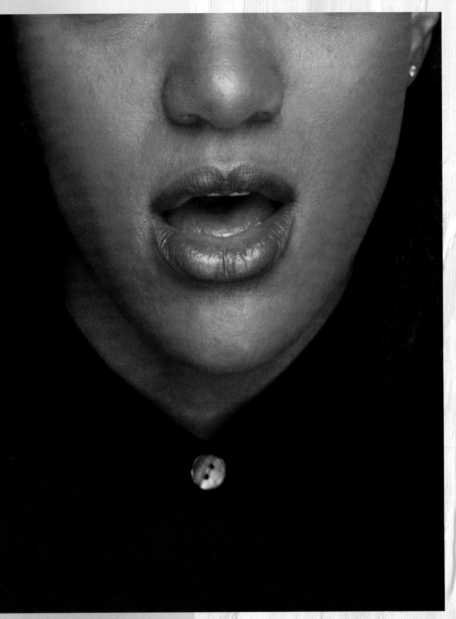

Above: allow your jaw to relax so that your mouth sags open.

sound is not spoken. No effort should be used to actually make a sound. Simply allow your out-breath to brush past your vocal cords, vibrating them as it goes. Stick with the 'Ah' sound and don't let it deteriorate into an 'Er', as this will require some effort.

12. As you finish exhaling, close your mouth.

13. Breathe in through your nose – steadily and controlled.

14. Go back to step 6 and repeat the process a further six times.

15. Remember to keep your breathing natural and rhythmic – and keep smiling.

As Alexander said 'There is a primary control of the use of the self which governs the working of all the mechanisms and so renders the control of the complex human organism comparatively simple'.

Only when these basics of the Alexander Technique have been mastered is it time to move on to more advanced techniques for situations that you will meet in every-day life.

10. Allow your jaw to relax so that your mouth sags open.

11. As you breathe out, whisper 'A-h-h-h-h-h-h'. This should be a long 'a' as in 'father'. Don't raise the level of the sound above a whisper, and let it begin as you start to exhale, and then fade as you finish breathing out. The

...But stay where you are for a moment and read on before you dash for your coffee.

Freeze – literally, just how you are at this moment. Don't move a muscle until you have finished answering the following questions:

How am I sitting (or standing)?

Would Alexander be proud to call me one of his pupils?

Is my neck free?

Is my head forwards and up?

Is my back lengthened and wide?

Am I breathing correctly?

Are the muscles that I am not using relaxed?

Is my body in a natural, comfortable position without any tension?

Finally – and most important – how did I come to be in this position?

Alexander considered these questions important and used them to form his hypothesis of 'the means whereby'. He described this as being the process of paying attention to 'the means whereby' an end – any end – is achieved. In this particular case we were looking at the means whereby you came to be in the position you were in when you started reading this section. Hence the last question.

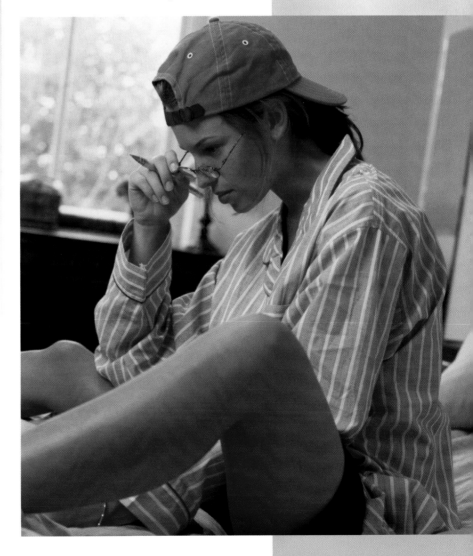

Below: is my body in a natural, comfortable position without any tension?

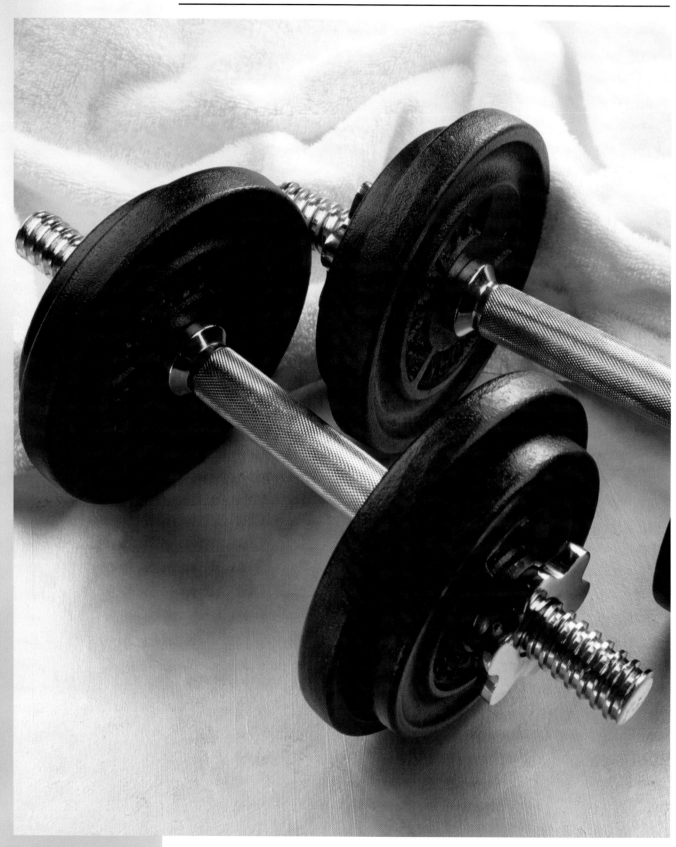

By using 'the means whereby' we can remove or reduce our bad habits. Alexander maintained that if we never thought about 'the means whereby', then we were acting out of habit, automatically. It is only when we make choices and begin to control our actions that we start to move as we should.

He followed up this idea by suggesting that we should 'stop before we start', which he called 'applied inhibition'. This meant stopping before we take any action and considering it before we carry it out in the correct manner. As Alexander put it, 'the conscious mind must be quickened'. Thus he taught himself to inhibit his natural way of speaking, consider his action and put into practice all that he had taught himself, before he ever opened his mouth.

Considering 'the means whereby', and stopping before you start may sound unnatural, but consider this: unless you apply this technique before picking up a heavy object from the floor, you may snatch it up without thinking. This could damage your back and/or rupture internal muscles and give you a hernia. Here is definitely a case where we must apply inhibition. As lifting is one of the things that most of us do wrongly – and without thinking – we will look at this in the next section.

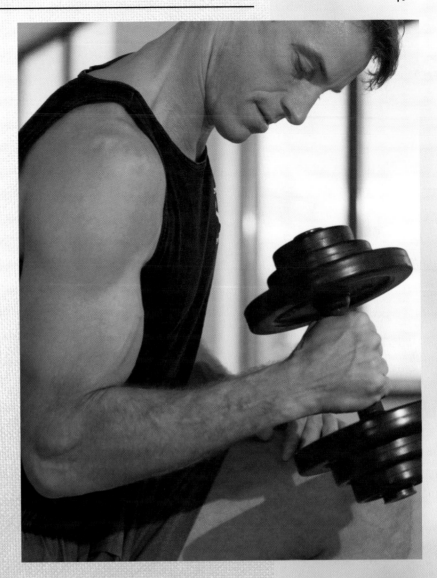

Above and left: 'applied inhibition' unless you apply this technique before picking up a heavy object from the floor, you may snatch it up without thinking. This could damage your back and/or rupture internal muscles and give you a hernia.

INDOORS

GETTING OUT OF BED

When you wake up in the morning I'm sure that you'll find it easy to stay in bed for a moment or two longer before leaping out. Most people like to defer that inevitable moment when they have to get up, and here is an excellent excuse.

If you are going to spend the day practising the Alexander Technique, this is the place to start.

Below: most people like to defer that inevitable moment when they have to get up.

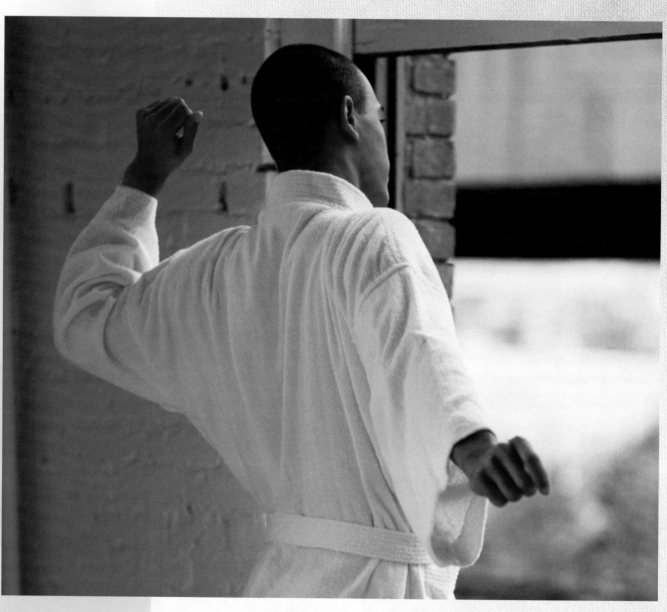

1. Lay on your back, legs straight, arms by your sides.

2. Take several breaths, ensuring that you apply the primary points of control.

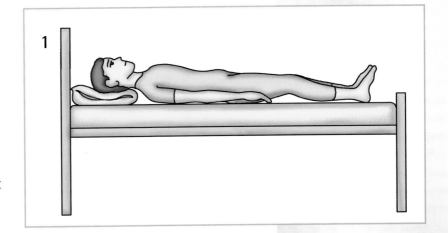

   a. Let your neck be free. Roll your head from side to side and circle it first one way and then the other.

   b. Push your head back into the pillow and then push your chin down to your chest before finally bringing it forwards and up.

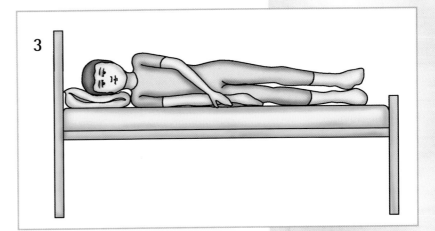

   c. Feel the muscles in your back as you allow it to lengthen and widen. At this point concentrate on the lengthening, as you have no weight on your back at this time.

3. Take another breath before you roll over on to your side, towards the side at which you will leave the bed.

4. Move your legs over the side of the bed.

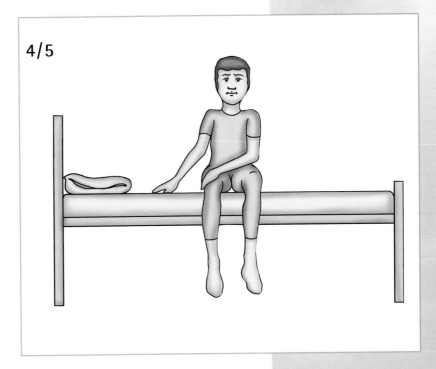

5. Push yourself into a sitting position by leaning forward, leading with your head.

6. Take another breath in before standing upright.

7. You are now ready to start the day.

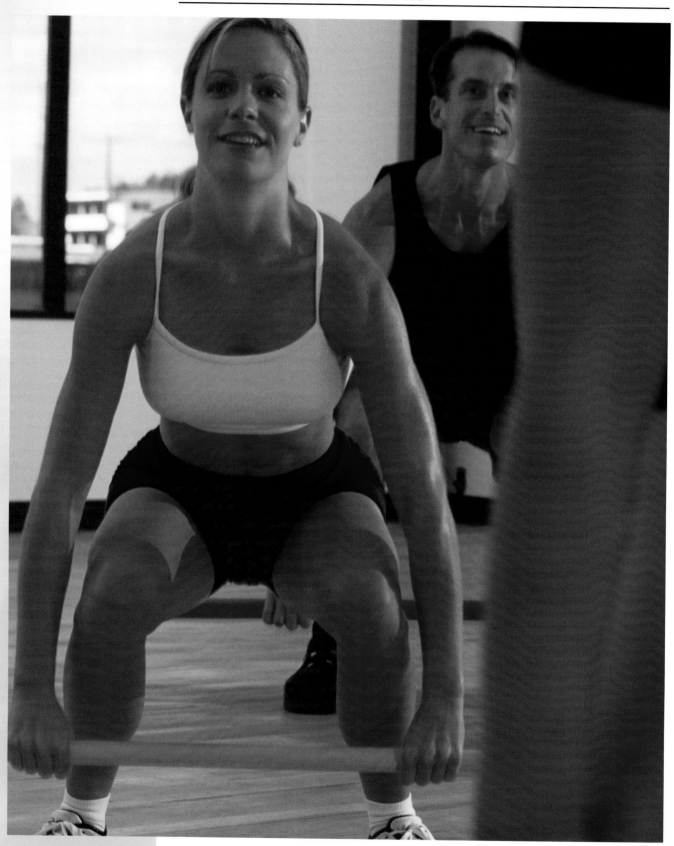

LIFTING

Using the wrong method of lifting heavy objects up from the floor is the main cause of many back problems and most hernias.

If you are to move an object that is on the floor, you must first bend and then lift before carrying, so we will look at these as three separate components. This technique is suitable for picking up anything from the floor, from getting a speck of dirt off the carpet to lifting a box full of books.

1. Place your feet at slightly less than shoulder width apart.

2. Make sure that your weight is equally distributed between both feet.

3. Allow your neck and shoulders to be free and relaxed.

4. Straighten and widen your back.

5. Let your head go forward.

6. Breathe out.

7. Bend – first from the ankles, then the knees.

8. Finally bend your body, from your hips, keeping your spine straight.

9. Pause for a moment to make sure that your neck, arms, shoulders and legs are not too tense.

10. Do not hold your breath.

11. Test the weight of the object to ensure that it is not going to be too heavy for you to lift on your own.

12. If it is within your capability, lift the object just clear of the floor.

13. Take another breath in.

14. Lean back so that the weight of the object is counterbalanced by your own body weight.

15. Straighten your knees and ankles.

16. Keep your arms as straight as possible without being stiff.

17. Only start to move once you are again upright, with your back perfectly straight and vertical.

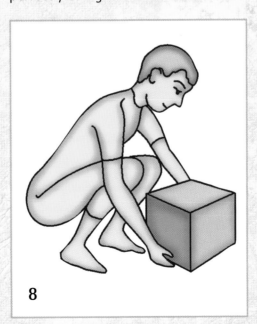

8

Far left: using the wrong method of lifting heavy objects up from the floor is the main cause of many back problems and most hernias. This stance you see has the feet too far apart and the head back intead of forward.

Below: when carrying heavy loads such as shopping or luggage, try to split your load into two equal amounts so that one can be carried in each hand, thus balancing the weight.

18. Take only small, steady steps, keeping the weight directly in front of you.

19. If you feel that you should rush to your destination because of the weight, put it back down and take a rest. Do not try to run carrying a heavy object.

20. When putting the object down, reverse the procedure of picking it up – back straight, ankles then knees and body bent.

21. Pause for a moment and take another breath before slowly standing upright.

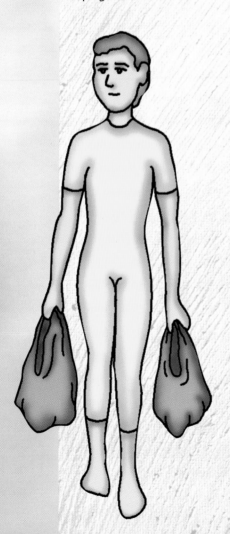

You will notice all the actual lifting is done with both the arms and the back straight. This will avoid any possibility of strain. The main muscles used are those in your thighs – the strongest muscles in the body. Do not be tempted to spread your legs further apart in order to get lower. It is when lifting from this position that a rupture of the internal musculature can occur.

If you are going to carry something – such as a suitcase – that will be carried on one side, again bend the knees before picking it off the ground. As you straighten up, try to keep your stance upright and don't let the weight pull your back over so that it is bent to the side. This happens when you think that by lowering the load, nearer to the ground, you are lessening the weight. This is not so, and twisting your back sideways will not only tire it more quickly, but also can lead to damage of the spine.

When carrying heavy loads such as shopping, try to split your purchases into two equal amounts so that one can be carried in each hand, thus balancing the weight. As you walk with this type of load, lean back slightly, thus keeping your back straight and upright, and shoulders loose, but back.

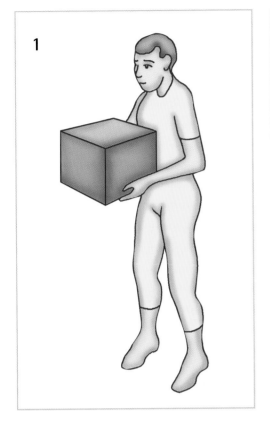

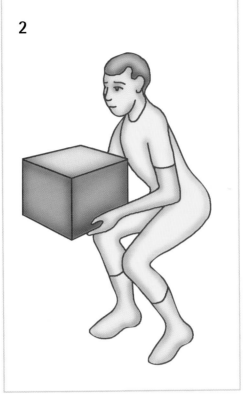

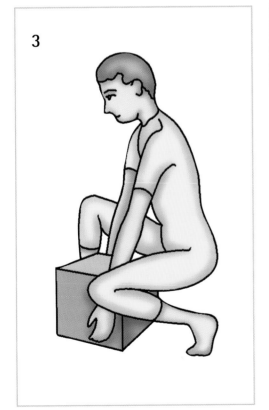

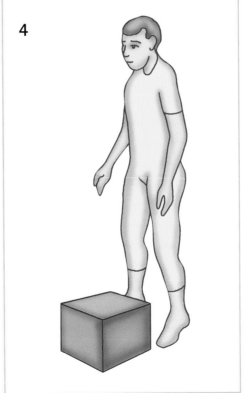

Left: when putting the object down, reverse the procedure of picking it up – back straight, ankles then knees and body bent.

READING

One of the most common posture errors that occur when sitting is made when you are reading. The reason for this is that, immersed in your book, you put all your thought into what you are reading and allow your body to relax. This usually means that you slouch in your chair and adopt a position that is bad for your back and your breathing.

To avoid making this mistake, use the following steps. And yes, that does apply to reading this book, too.

1. Sit on your chair in a comfortable position with both feet flat on the floor.

2. Avoid being tense. Relax sufficiently to allow the back of the chair to support your lower spine.

3. Check that you are sitting so that your weight is evenly distributed on both sides of your pelvis.

4. Lift your book so that it is at a comfortable height and reading distance.

5. Allow your neck to relax and fall forward slightly so that you are looking straight at the book.

6. Hold the book so that it is angled to your body, and the pages are square to your line of vision.

7. Use one hand to support the book and the other to keep the pages open. Using this method you will not be tempted to grip the book, as you may well do otherwise, especially if the story is exciting.

8. If you are reading an exceptionally large or heavy book, rest it on a desk, propped up so that it is at a convenient height and angle, resembling a lectern.

9. Occasionally rest the book back down on your lap. This will allow your arms to relax and let you change your focus as you look away.

10. However exciting the book, remember to keep breathing steadily and correctly.

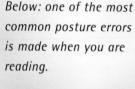

Below: one of the most common posture errors is made when you are reading.

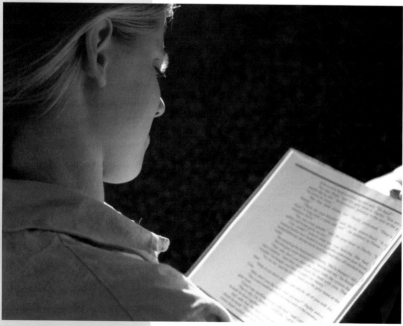

WRITING

The most important factor for establishing a good posture when writing is to have the desk top at the correct height relative to your chair. The only way, usually, is to adjust your chair to bring you to the correct level.

Adjust your seated height so that your elbows are level with the desk top. This means that you should be able to lay your forearm flat on the desk.

It is important to spend some time getting this just right if you are going to be writing for more than a short time.

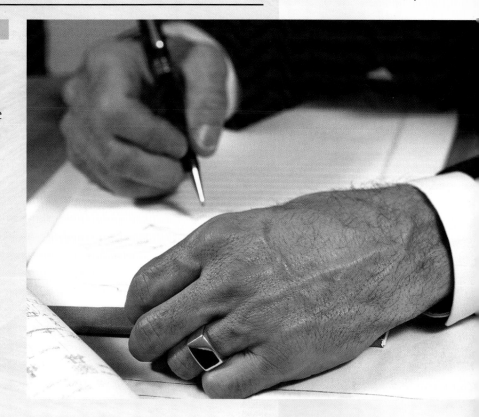

Above: when writing only grip the pen as much as is necessary to control it.

1. Pull your chair towards the desk so that you can comfortably rest your wrists on the edge of it without having to reach forward or pull your elbows back.

2. Lay your hands flat on the desk, shoulder width apart.

3. Relax your neck so that you can look down easily.

4. Take a breath in and then out.

5. Stretch your fingers forward.

6. Turn your hands over so that the back of them rests on the desk.

7. Take another complete breath.

8. Stretch your fingers again.

9. Turn your hands back so that your palms are flat on the desk again.

10. Lift your hands up by flexing your wrists while keeping your wrists on the desk.

11. Keeping your palms flat on the desk, lift your fingers and thumbs up as far as possible so as to stretch them.

12. Open your shoulders.

13. Take up your pen and allow your other hand to rest flat on the desk at shoulder width from your writing hand.

Right: most writing these days is done not with a pen, but at a keyboard.

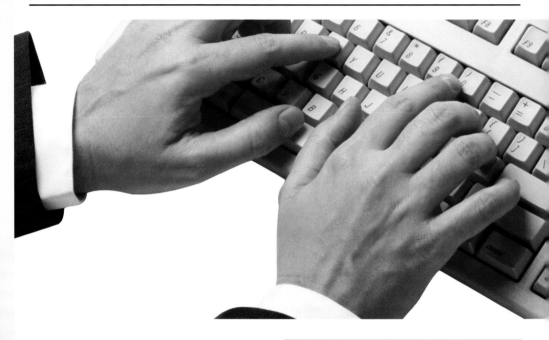

USING A KEYBOARD

14. Keep your spine straight. Avoid the temptation to lean forward over your writing, so that your nose gets ever closer to the paper. If you do have to lean forward, you are not seated correctly.

15. Only grip the pen as much as is necessary to control it.

16. To avoid writer's cramp take frequent breaks. One good idea is to give yourself a rest at the end of every page. Put your pen down and flex the fingers and thumb of your writing hand, stretching and then relaxing them.

Most writing these days is done not with a pen, but at a keyboard. The modern keyboard is much kinder than the old-fashioned typewriter. You no longer have to pound the keys, as you did previously, nor do you have to lift your hands up to the keyboard. The modern keyboard is so flat and level that you can sit at it as though you were going to write.

Nevertheless, many problems have been experienced by those who work at keyboards for long periods. Most of these could have been prevented if the operator had known about and used the Alexander Technique.

1. Sit as before, with your chair an inch (25mm) or so higher than you had it for writing, so that this time your elbows are level in height with the keys.

2. Move your chair so that when your fingers are on the mid row of keys – the 'home' position for your hands – your upper arm is vertical.

3. Sit for a moment and relax, but ensure that you remember and apply the primary points of control:

Let the neck be free.

Let the head go forwards and up.

Allow the back to lengthen and widen.

4. Notice where your gaze comes to rest. This will usually be slightly lower than level with the horizon. Any monitor you are viewing should have its centre at this level. Tilt the monitor so that its axis is square to your line of vision.

5. Ensure that the screen is at a convenient distance for you to see it clearly without eye-strain.

6. Keep your shoulders relaxed and open as you type.

7. If you are copy-typing, make sure that your copy is easily visible without having to strain your neck to read it. If possible, use a copy-holder alongside your monitor. Also make certain that the copy is well lit so that you do not have to lean forward to peer at it.

8. Keep your wrists relaxed. Use a wrist-pad if you can and rest your wrists on it between periods of keying in – such as when pausing to read from the monitor.

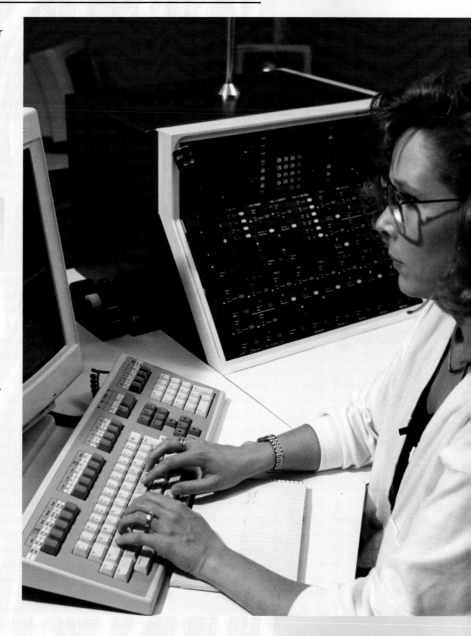

Above: many problems have been experienced by those who work at keyboards for long periods. Most of these could have been prevented if the operator had known about and used the Alexander Technique.

9. If possible, zoom in on the writing or numbers that appear on your screen so that, as before, you do not have to lean forward to read them clearly and easily. If you do need to take a closer look at the screen occasionally, remember to bend forward from the hips, rather than craning your neck. Remember to return to an upright position before you resume using your keyboard.

10. Take frequent breaks, even if you remain at the keyboard. Look away from the monitor, drop your arms to your sides and shake your hands with the wrists and fingers relaxed and loose. Look around from side to side so as to loosen your neck muscles.

11. Take a complete break every half-hour. Get up, walk away from your desk and take five minutes before returning to work. If you are in the habit of getting so involved in your work that you forget time altogether, try this. Shift everything off your desk except your keyboard, mouse, monitor and CPU. Now, whenever you need to use a notepad, pencil, dictionary, reference book or anything else, you will have to get up and leave your desk, i.e. take a break.

12. If you don't touch-type, consider taking a course. Continually looking down to the keyboard and then back to the monitor means that your neck is working overtime – with potentially disastrous results.

Below: take a complete break every half-hour. Get up, walk away from your desk and take five minutes before returning to work. Remember to return to an upright position before you resume using your keyboard.

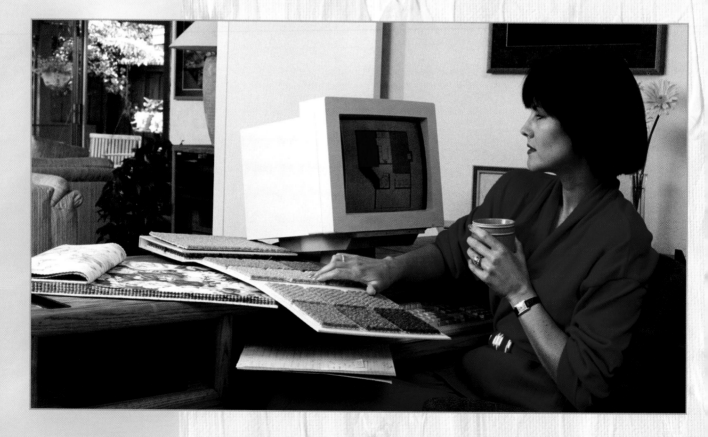

MONKEY

F. M. Alexander perfected a technique of standing and bending that he called 'a position of mechanical advantage'. His pupils took one look at the position he had taken and promptly christened it 'monkey', and so it has been called ever since. Once you have adopted this position, you will immediately see why. 'Monkey' is a stance in which your muscles are relaxed and at the same time the various parts of your body are in alignment.

There is an easy way to check your alignment and at the same time obtain the perfect monkey stance. This little exercise, for obvious reasons, is called 'monkey against a wall':

1. Wear loose clothing and no footwear at all.

2. Stand with your back to a smooth wall. (This is important, as you will have to slide down it later on. If no suitable wall is available, a smooth-panelled door will serve just as well.)

3. Take up a position where your feet are shoulder width apart and your heels 2 inches (5cm) away from the wall.

4. Allow your hands and arms to hang loosely by your side.

5. Stand upright, remembering, as ever, to apply the primary points of control:

> *Let the neck be free.*
> *Let the head go forwards and up.*
> *Allow the back to lengthen and widen.*

6. If you are standing correctly, you will not be touching the wall at this time. If you are touching it, straighten up and lean away from it until you are balanced and not in contact with it at any point.

7. Breathe in, and at the same time allow your weight to go back on your heels so that you lean lightly against the wall.

Below: stand with your back to a smooth wall. Breathe in, and at the same time allow your weight to go back on your heels so that you lean lightly against the wall.

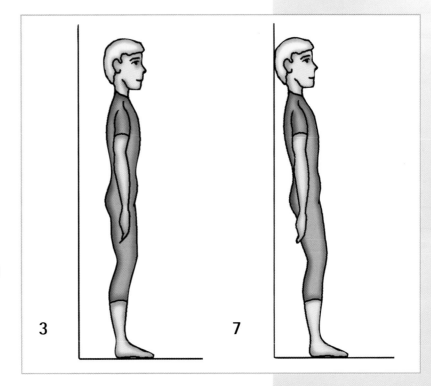

3   7

8. Stop immediately when you feel the first point of contact has been made.

9. If you are well aligned, you will note that your two shoulders and your buttocks have all touched the wall at the same time. If they didn't, you are not properly aligned. Note whether:

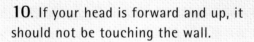

Your pelvis is too far back (if your buttocks alone touch the wall).

Your pelvis is too far forward (if your shoulders touch first).

Your spine is twisted (if one shoulder only touches the wall.)

10. If your head is forward and up, it should not be touching the wall.

11. Adjust your position so that you can feel the four points of contact – both shoulders and both buttocks evenly pressed against the wall.

12. With one hand check the space between your lower back and the wall. You will probably find a gap into which you can push your hand.

13. To eliminate this gap, bend your knees slightly and allow your ankles to flex so that your shoulders and pelvis start to slide down the wall. Keep your four points in contact with the wall and let your hands and arms hang by your side.

14. You are now in the correct position of mechanical advantage – a perfect monkey position.

15. This is the way to bend down when about to pick up something from the floor. If your shoulders come away from the wall as you do this, you are bending forward, as most people do.

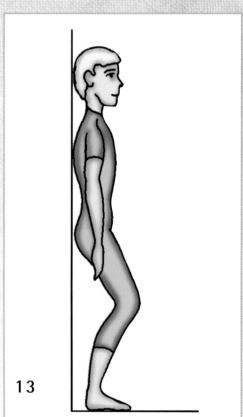

13

Below: if you are well aligned, you will note that your two shoulders and your buttocks have all touched the wall at the same time.

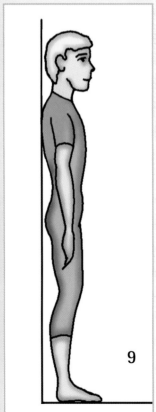

9

16. Try to maintain this position as you walk a few steps away from the wall. You will have to lean forward before you can do this, but keep your spine straight. This is how monkeys walk and is mid-way between the way we moved several million years ago and how we walk today. It has now become difficult and unnatural for us to move about like this – but note that your body is balanced and in perfect alignment.

17. Return to the wall and finish off by sliding back up until you are once again standing upright. You should be able to do this without any pressure on the wall and without the use of any muscles other than those in your thighs that allow you to straighten your knees.

If your body is out of alignment, you may find it tiring to stand in the monkey position for any length of time. Resolve to continue practising until it becomes easier and more natural to you. Once you do this, you will find that posture has improved and both movement and poise will take much less effort.

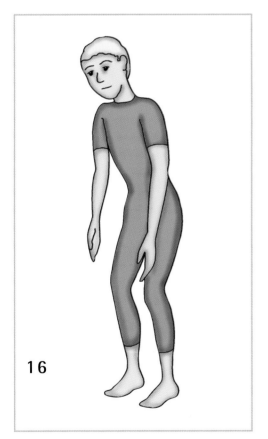

16

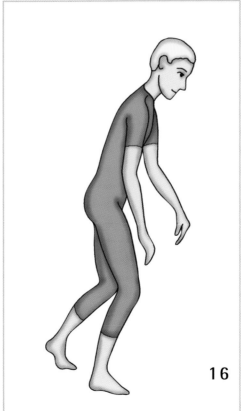

16

Left: try to maintain this position as you walk a few steps away from the wall. You will have to lean forward before you can do this, but keep your spine straight. This is how monkeys walk and is mid-way between the way we moved several million years ago and how we walk today.

OUT AND ABOUT

DRIVING A CAR

One of the most common outdoor activities these days is driving a car. Driving for any length of time will tire your body and this leads to mental fatigue. The combination of mental and physical exhaustion can have catastrophic results, from road rage to falling asleep at the wheel. Though the Alexander Technique can help you to relax while driving and thus delay fatigue, it cannot be over-emphasised that every long journey should be punctuated with proper breaks away from the vehicle.

Unfortunately we were not born to drive – it is not a skill that comes naturally, like standing and walking. We have to learn, and although we are taught the actual skill of manoeuvring and controlling the vehicle, nobody ever thinks to teach us how to do it with minimum effort and stress. For this reason, driving is the greatest cause of lower back pain, and consequent absence from work. Long-haul drivers are also three times more likely to have disc problems than anyone else.

By applying the Alexander Technique you will find even the most arduous journey less tiring, less stressful and therefore safer.

1. Before you can start driving you have to get into the car. After you have opened the door, turn your back to the car, bend your back and lower your bottom onto the seat.

2. Then swing round, lifting both legs and feet, keeping them together.

3. Once you are sitting facing forward, lift your bottom again so that you can push the base of your spine as far back as it will go into the seat.

Below: driving for any length of time will tire your body and this leads to mental fatigue.

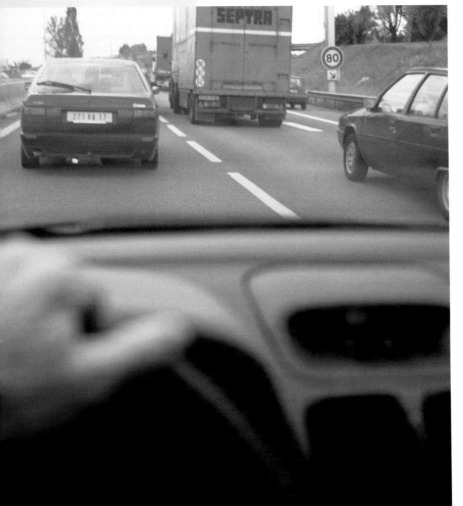

4. Take hold of the steering wheel at the quarter-to-two position and put your left foot on the clutch pedal. Depress this pedal as far as is needed to change gear.

5. Check that:

Your arms are slightly bent at the elbow. Avoid a straight-arm position where the elbows are locked.

Your foot rests comfortably on the pedal and you have not had to stretch or twist to the left in order to depress it completely.

You are not crouched, head forward, to peer through the windscreen.

You are not gripping the steering wheel for a 'white knuckle' ride. Relax your wrists as well as your hands.

Your back is fully supported from your shoulders to the base of your spine.

6. If necessary, move the seat position and add supplementary support until you are sure that you can answer all the above points in the affirmative.

7. Put your seat belt on and now make sure that you maintain the correct driving position.

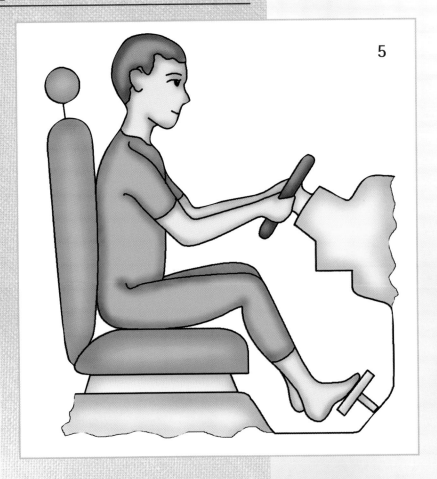

8. As you sit in the car, remember to apply the primary points of control:

Let the neck be free.

Let the head go forwards and up.

Allow the back to lengthen and widen.

9. Before you set off, check your driving mirror again. It may need adjustment as a result of your improved posture.

Above: a good driving posture.

10. Try to stay relaxed as you drive, while remaining alert. Be aware of the slightest amount of tension that creeps into your body due to any stress.

11. Take every opportunity to rest while you are still in the driving seat. This may be while held up in a traffic jam, waiting at the traffic lights, or even while you are waiting to move out at a junction. In these odd moments move your head from side to side to relax your neck muscles. Take your hands off the wheel, drop them to your sides and shake them from the wrists.

12. Draw your feet back so that you can rest them, even momentarily, flat on the floor. Make sure that you have the handbrake on and that you are out of gear when you do this.

13. While the car is stationary, lift your bottom from the seat and push back. After any length of time driving it is almost certain that your body will have slumped somewhat.

Below: a bad driving posture.

14. As you drive along there will be periods of time when you can become conscious of your posture.
Try to make it a habit of checking it every so often as you drive. Just ask yourself:

Am I staying relaxed? Note whether you are clenching your jaw.

Am I gripping the steering wheel too tightly? Note whether your knuckles are white.

Have I forgotten the primary control points? Check to see if your neck muscles are taut.

Have I slumped down in my seat? Notice whether you need to push your spine back so that it is supported correctly.

15. When reversing, release your seat belt. (This is the only time that it is legal to do so when you are driving .) Taking off your seat belt allows you to turn the whole of your upper body so that you are not twisting your neck to an uncomfortable degree.

16. Finally, when you arrive at your destination, take just as much care getting out of the car as you did getting in. Open the door, swing both feet out until they are flat on the ground, bend your back and lean forward until your weight is over your feet and you can stand upright.

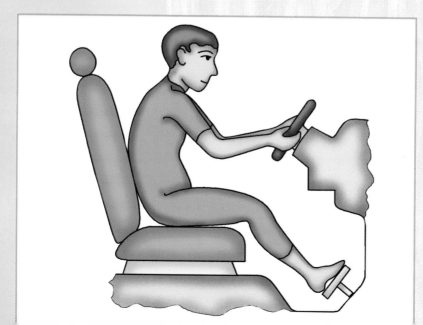

RIDING A BICYCLE

Cycle riding can be a relaxing mode of transport as well as a healthy way of getting about in the fresh air. At the same time it also exercises many of the body's muscles. So cycling is good for you – but there are a few qualifications. If the cycle is not set up correctly – which means set up specifically for you – or if you do not ride it properly, then you can do more damage than good. Cyclists, like motorists, can do immeasurable harm to their backs if these points are not heeded.

First, is this the right size bike for you? Cycle frames come in different sizes and there is a correct size for you. Choose one that is too big and you may find it impossible to ride with any control at all. We have all seen youngsters attempting to ride their big brother's bike, wobbling from side to side as they try to maintain contact with the pedals. Choose one that is too small and you will find your knees hitting your forearms or you will have to ride with your knees brought up outside your arms; both of which are highly unstable and dangerous ways to ride.

Several adjustments can be made to tailor the bike to your requirements.

Below: cycle riding can be a relaxing mode of transport as well as a healthy way of getting about in the fresh air.

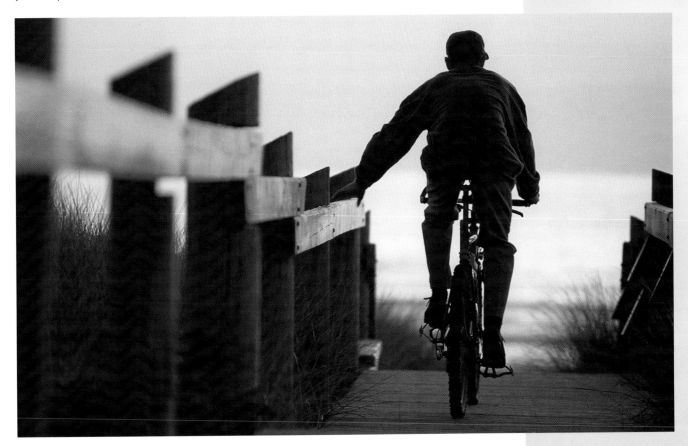

1. The height of the saddle. Adjust this so that when you are sitting comfortably you can touch the ground with the tips of both feet at the same time.

2. The angle of the saddle. This should be fixed to give maximum support when pedalling. If it is tipped back too much, it will be extremely uncomfortable; if tipped forward, you will tend to slide forward.

3. The height of the handlebars is important as this determines the angle of your spine and neck. Sit on the bike and hold the handlebars. Now look ahead. If your neck is strained or your back bowed, then the handlebars should be raised. If you are leaning too far forward, your elbows will be braced to take your weight. You will tire very quickly as well as put considerable strain on your shoulders.

Below: mountain bikes have been designed for off-road use, on rough terrain where the rider has no use for a saddle.

4. The angle of the handlebars should be adjusted so that the grips fall naturally into your hands without flexing the wrists. When you grip the handlebars there should be equal pressure across your palm.

5. As you ride along, your legs, ankles and feet are the only parts of your body that should be moving. You should still be able to maintain the primary points of control with your neck free, your head forwards and up, and your back lengthened and wide. Unless you are using your cycle for racing, stick to this set-up.

6. A cycle for racing is assembled so that when the rider is mounted, his body presents the least resistance to the air. An aerodynamic shape is necessary for maximum speed with no thought to the tension, stress or discomfort of the rider.

A final note is necessary about the mountain bike, which is a different kettle of fish. These bikes have been designed for off-road use, on rough terrain where the rider has no use for a saddle. Unfortunately they have now become a cult item and are ridden on our roads. It is impossible to ride these cycles and maintain Alexander's primary position as they can only be ridden with the weight thrown forward, neck strained and excessive pressure on the ankles.

Do be sure that you buy the correct cycle for your specific needs.

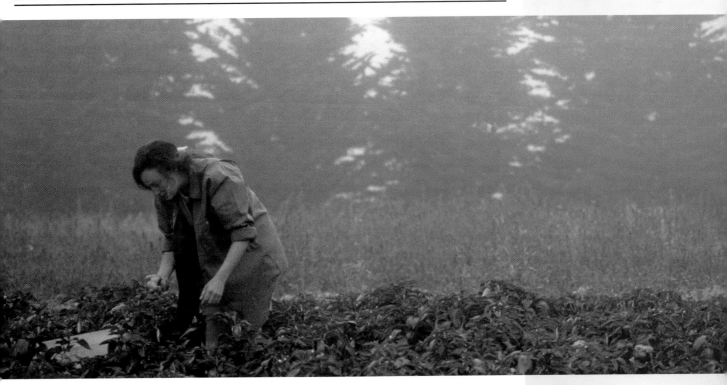

GARDENING

Another area in which the Alexander Technique is useful is to help maintain good posture and thus prevent damage when gardening.

We have all seen pictures of the weekend gardener, trying to straighten up his back with one hand while leaning on his spade with the other. It is often not realised just how much damage you can do to yourself in the garden. Here you push, pull, stretch, crouch, reach and lift far more than you do when working indoors. In all these actions you will benefit from application of the Alexander Technique.

Alexander himself maintained that his technique could be compared to gardening – noting that there were no satisfactory short-cuts in either.

One of the problems that stems from gardening is that most people do it only periodically and the greatest effort has to be made after the longest rest. Hence when you turn over the garden in the spring you use muscles that have not been exercised for many months, and end up suffering from back pains.

Here is a chance to apply some of the lessons learned indoors. For a start there is usually lots of bending and picking up from the ground to be done. If necessary, go back to the section on LIFTING and read it again before going any further.

Above: one of the problems with gardening is that most people do it only periodically.

USING A WHEELBARROW

1. Lifting is one thing, carrying another. For moving all but the lightest loads, use a wheelbarrow. You will, quite naturally by now, have kept your spine straight while bending to pick up and place your load in the wheelbarrow.

2. To pick up the barrow, keep your spine upright, let your neck be free, let your head go forwards and up.

3. Bend from the knees and ankles, allowing your back to lengthen and widen.

4. Grasp the handles and straighten your legs, making sure that you keep your arms straight. Avoid snatching the barrow up and trying to use the muscles of your arms to help.

5. Lean forward and, as the barrow starts to move, follow it. This sounds very simplistic, but the point is to avoid pushing the barrow with any force. This would cause a lot of work for your back muscles and possibly strain them.

6. At the end of your journey, lower the barrow by bending your knees again until it touches the ground.

Below: for moving all but the lightest loads, use a wheelbarrow.

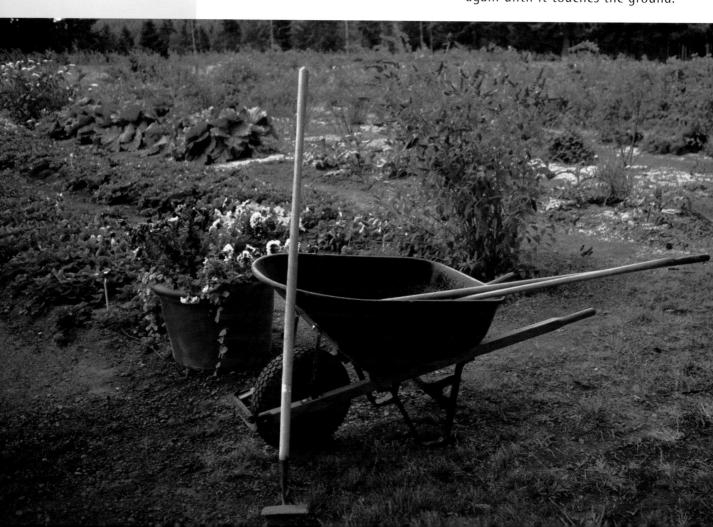

DIGGING

Digging can be tiring. The speed at which you tire will depend on at least three factors – the size of the spade, the type of soil, and finally your method – to say nothing of your general state of fitness.

Choose a spade that you know is not too heavy for you to handle over a short period of time. Avoid using a shovel that is used for shifting quantities of loose material by builders and navvies rather than gardeners.

The soil we can do nothing about, but you can apply the Alexander Technique to help you dig more easily:

1. Stand in an upright position. Don't try to push the spade into the ground so as to lift too much soil.

2. Use your weight, through your foot, to push the spade into the ground. Avoid trying to use your body weight through your hands to press the spade down. At this point there is no need to grip the spade tightly.

3. Lean back, pulling on the spade handle to loosen the soil.

4. Bend your knees and use your body as a counterweight as you lift the spadeful of soil.

5. Move your lower hand down the spade shaft as you lift and try to keep this arm straight.

6. Move forward before turning the spade over to empty it, rather than trying to throw the soil. Throwing the soil exerts terrific and sudden stress on the back muscles that can easily be torn by such a movement.

7. If this is done correctly, you should be able to keep your spine straight at all times as the bending should come from the hips.

8. Rest frequently, especially if you are not used to this form of exercise.

Below: choose a spade that you know is not too heavy.

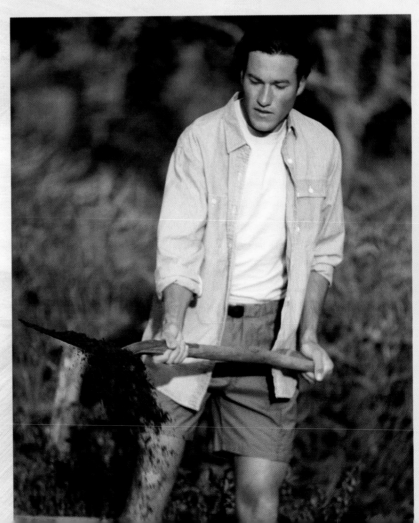

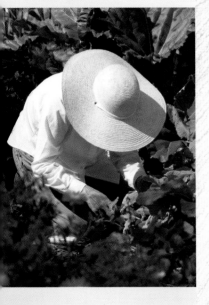

Below: some garden jobs are best done on your knees.

WEEDING

Some garden jobs, and weeding is one of them, are best done on your knees. But not many people enjoy being on their knees for any length of time. The reason is that our knees are not designed to take our weight in the way that they have to when kneeling down. Use the following technique and you will not find it as tiring:

1. Before you start, get something to kneel on. An old mat or folded sack is ideal. Also, wear gardening gloves.

2. Get down by bending from the knees, ankles and hips, keeping the back straight.

3. As you settle down with your weight on your knees, lean further forward from the hips and rest both hands on the ground in front of you.

4. Allow the weight of your upper body to be taken on your hands.

5. Apply the primary points of control: i.e. let the neck be free; let the head go forwards and up; allow the back to lengthen and widen.

6. As much as possible, use one hand for weeding, taking the weight of your upper body on the other. This takes a great deal of your weight off your knees and allows you to work longer without tiring.

7. Aim to work a short distance in front of the hand you are resting on, so that you are reaching forward. This ensures that your head remains forward and up as you look ahead to where you are weeding.

8. Occasionally alternate which hand you are weeding with and which hand you rest on.

9. Take frequent breaks. Stand up using the technique learned earlier:

While still on all fours, slowly rock backwards and forwards until you can sit back on your heels.

From this position push yourself up and bring one leg forward.

Rest again in this crouched position. Keep your body upright, push up on the forward leg and bring your other leg alongside to regain a full standing position.

Stand for a moment and take a couple of deep breaths before moving off.

10. Move around, rather than standing to take your rest, and keep moving until you feel that your knees are ready to let you kneel down again.

SWEEPING UP

If you do need to kneel down, it's a good idea to have another job in the garden to alternate with the weeding. Make sure that this is one that you can do while standing upright – such as pruning or mowing the lawn. Then you won't feel that you are wasting your time when taking a break from weeding. It will also ensure that you take a longer break between sessions of kneeling than you would have done otherwise.

Inevitably after gardening there is some sweeping up to be done. Even if care has been taken with the rest of the gardening, it all can be undone if you don't think what you are doing when sweeping. Inevitably all jobs take longer than anticipated, so you rush the last bit. Don't! Take the following steps:

1. Take hold of the brush lightly. Avoid gripping it more tightly than necessary.

2. Allow the weight of the brush, as much as is possible, to be all that is needed to do the sweeping. In other words, don't press down on the brush any more than is needed.

3. If you apply the primary points of control with your neck free, your head forwards and up, and allow your back to lengthen and widen, you will find that you do not need to use the strength of your arms so much.

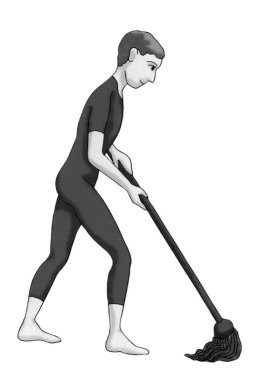

4. As you step forward, use that motion to do the sweeping, using the muscular power of your back and your legs, rather than your arms. This will ensure that you maintain a good posture and you will not find it at all tiring.

TAKE A BREAK: 3

TAKING EXERCISE

We are all aware of the importance of exercise, and many people undertake some activity regularly – say on a daily or weekly basis. You may be taking vigorous exercise, such as playing squash, or some more gentle form, such as T'ai Chi. You may prefer a solitary pursuit for your work-out or practise a group sport. Also you may be taking your exercise either indoors or out. Whichever form of exercise you take, the principles and the practice – as far as Alexander Technique are concerned – are the same.

If we do exercise, it is usually to keep our body fit. And we keep fit to enable us to carry out the everyday tasks of our daily lives more easily and with less fatigue. Exercising is a conscious task that we undertake voluntarily. So it should be something that we enjoy. This is fulfilled most commonly by sports where there is some competitive edge to add to the enjoyment.

There is no point in gritting your teeth and hating every moment of your undertaking. You will end up doing more harm than good, or giving up all together. Your exercise should be a form of recreation in both its present and former meanings – 'refreshing and entertaining', as well as 'restoring to a good or wholesome condition' – literally 're-creation'.

Similarly, don't feel that you will benefit from exhausting yourself at your exercise. It has been shown that 'the burn-out' is counter-productive and dangerous. When you feel that you have had enough, stop. Never go as far as the pain barrier. Always leave a little energy in reserve.

As exercise is mainly a physical activity, there is usually plenty of time for thought. Employ at least some of that time to consider how you can apply the principles of the Alexander Technique to what you are doing.

If you can, occasionally throughout your activity, bring to mind the primary points of control.

Let the neck be free.

Let the head go forwards and up.

Allow the back to lengthen and widen.

All vigorous exercise is designed to increase the body's oxygen intake. This means that we need to breathe deeper and more frequently – that is why we pant when taking vigorous exercise. If you apply the three primary points, your breathing will be easier, your oxygen intake greater and you will be able to release more energy into your exercise.

END-GAINING

F. M. Alexander made another point that is appropriate here. He coined the term 'end-gaining' to describe the process of focusing so much on the end result of whatever we are doing that we fail to take care of how that result is obtained.

A typical example of this can occur when we run. At first, remembering Alexander's primary points, you feel that your running is comfortable and easy, so you decide to speed up – have a little sprint, perhaps just as far as the next tree. What happens? You forget what you are doing and how you are doing it, and instead concentrate on your goal. You tense yourself up, grit your teeth and pound the ground. You flail with your arms and tuck your head down. You start to gasp for breath. You become an utter disaster. Why? Because you were end-gaining, which – as you realised when looking back – was detrimental to achieving your goal.

One of the best all-round exercises there is, and to which the Alexander Technique can be applied to good effect, is swimming. Here your body can relax in the water without gravity pulling you down. While swimming or floating you can lengthen your back to its fullest extent, as it doesn't have to support the weight of your upper body, arms

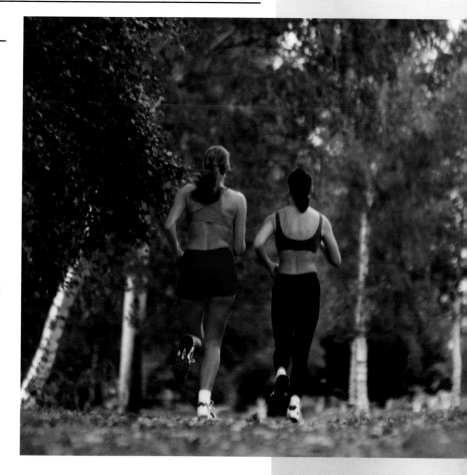

and head. Take full advantage of this opportunity to loosen up your back and neck muscles by floating for a short time. Become aware of your spine and consciously allow it to relax. As you swim you will find a new freedom in the water that allows you to move your body in the most natural way without straining any muscles.

If you are employed in a sedentary occupation and don't take any form of regular exercise, I suggest for your own well-being that you do so. And if you do, remember that there is no better starting point than swimming.

Above: a typical example of end-gaining can occur when we run.

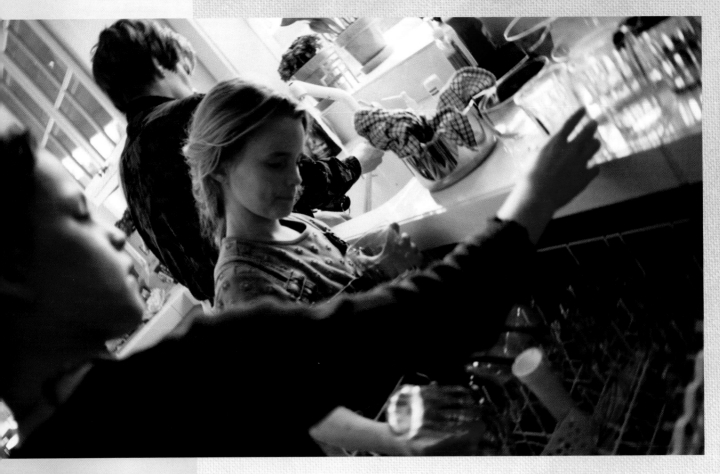

Above: you tend to do housework on 'automatic pilot'.

BACK INDOORS

EVERYDAY HOUSEHOLD ACTIVITIES

Inevitably, as much as we dislike doing it, there are a lot of jobs to be done about the house that are classed as 'housework'. The advantage of housework is that while you get on with the dusting you can let your mind relax. But because of this mental relaxation you will tend to do your jobs 'on automatic pilot'. You then forget about what you are doing with your body, and end up with poor posture and stress.

If we look at just a few of these jobs as examples, you'll be able to see how to use the Alexander Technique to improve your general well-being while undertaking these chores.

As you know, the main premise is to apply Alexander's primary points of control: let the neck be free; let the head go forwards and up; and allow the back to lengthen and widen. As long as you remember this primary control at all times, you will not go far wrong.

USING THE VACUUM CLEANER

Most people do not enjoy using a vacuum cleaner. It is noisy and it is heavy to push and to pull. Fortunately some far-sighted manufacturers have at last realised this and are now producing quieter, lighter models.

But this is no consolation for the thousands of owners of older models. The following technique will make it much less tiring and stressful:

1. Keep the vacuum cleaner in a cupboard where it is easy to get at. Avoid having to lift it out.

2. As with all appliances, hold it using no more grip than is necessary.

3. Wheel it to where you wish to use it. All vacuum cleaners wheel easily and there should be no need to carry it.

4. As you start to move it, lean forward so that your body weight is used to push the cleaner. Tilt the handle so that your weight pushes down through it to move the cleaner along. Don't try to push it from a standing position using only your arms. This puts considerable strain on your back.

5. Keep your neck free, allow your head to go forwards and up, and lengthen and widen your back.

6. When you wish to pull the vacuum cleaner back, do so by leaning away from it, so that it is bound to follow you. Your weight is sufficient to pull the cleaner back. Don't use your arm muscles. This would cause even more strain on your back.

7. Try to set up a regular tempo, not only with your movement of the cleaner but with your breathing as well. Once you find a suitable rhythm of breathing, pushing and pulling, you will find the whole operation much easier.

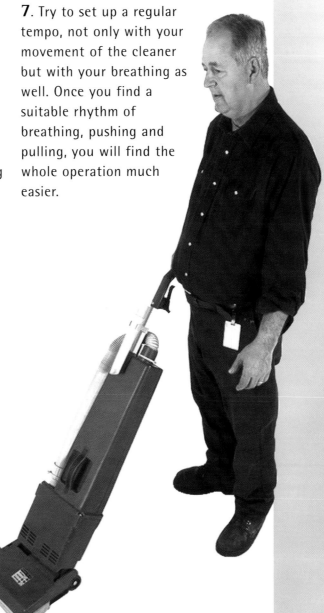

Below: most people do not enjoy using a vacuum cleaner.

SEWING

This activity is one that is usually undertaken in the sitting position, and as this has already been covered there should be no problem here.

The main point is to remember to keep your shoulders open. There is a tendency to rest your sewing on your lap and peer at it with closed shoulders, a bent back and lowered head.

Below: sewing is usually undertaken in the sitting position.

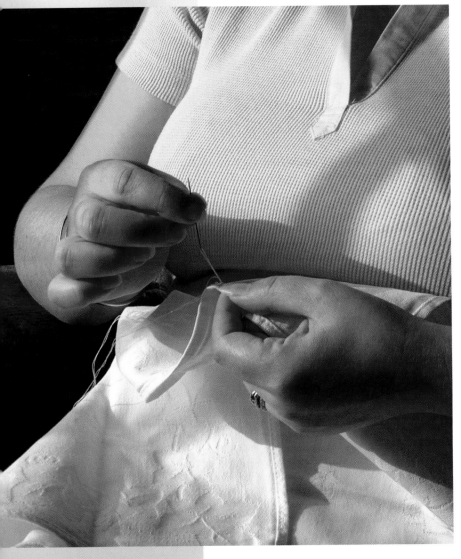

1. Lift the sewing up as you do when reading a book, until it is at a comfortable distance to see without bending over.

2. If anything, lean back. If you sit in an upright chair, make sure that you are supported at the base of your spine as well as at the shoulders.

3. If you start by consciously resting back, your spine will be straight, and if supported correctly it will also be relaxed.

4. Occasionally make a conscious check that you have remained in an upright position.

As with everything else, it's all a matter of practice. If you have always kept your sewing on your lap and bent over it, you will find it will take some time to break the habit. But with perseverance you will find that – because sitting correctly is also less tiring – you will pay more attention to maintaining a good posture and allow that to become your new habit.

IRONING

Ironing can be tiring for several reasons – including the obvious ones of heat and having to stand. But ask yourself if you do have to stand. With the ironing board at the correct height and a chair to suit, ironing can be done sitting down.

But if you prefer to stand up, make sure that you do it correctly:

1. Ensure that you have your ironing board at the correct height.

2. Check this by standing up to it with the iron flat on the board, as it will be when you are using it. Adjust the height of the board to that the iron's handle is level with your elbows when you let your arms hang naturally at your side.

3. Stand at the board in the natural stance, with your weight equally distributed between your two feet.

4. Only grip the iron as much as is necessary to pick it up and move it.

5. As ever, let your neck relax, let your head go forwards and up, and remember to lengthen and widen your back.

6. Although irons are lighter than they used to be, there is usually no need to press down on them and exert any force as you move the iron.

7. Instead, allow the iron to glide over the material at a slightly slower pace. You will get the same result as you did previously when you moved it quickly over the material while pushing down.

8. Check occasionally to see that your back is still straight. The tendency is to gradually lean over the ironing board. Your ironing may take a little longer, but you will find it much less tiring and much less stressful to the back.

With all household activities there is always a hard way and an easy way to accomplish the task. If you apply the Alexander Technique to them, you will find that they are less tiring and stressful.

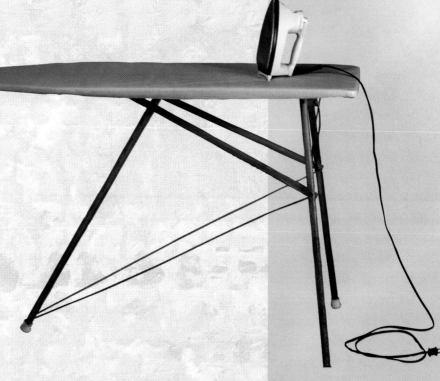

Below: ironing can be tiring for several reasons.

Far right: standing at a sink and washing dishes can be tiring.

WASHING-UP

Standing at a sink and washing dishes can be tiring as it is one of the few cases where we can adjust neither the height of our working surface, nor our own position.

The easy way out is to use a dish-washer, but space or economics may prevent you from being able to do this.

There are two ways in which the job can be made easier, if you have to do it by hand. The first is to use the Alexander Technique.

1. Stand in the controlled relaxed position. This usually means that you have to lean forward to reach into the sink. If this is so, keep your spine straight, though bent forward and at the same time bend your knees slightly so that they are not braced back. If your knees strike the cupboard door that usually boxes the sink in, open it and try again.

2. Remember to apply the primary points of control:

Let your neck be free, though your head will be bent forward to see what you are doing.

Let your head go forwards and up as much as possible. In other words, don't let your chin rest on your chest and restrict your breathing.

Allow your back to lengthen and widen. This is of vital importance as the tendency is to close your shoulders, which again hampers your breathing.

3. Try to remain relaxed and not tensed up. Think about this so that you will be conscious of any tension that you can then immediately counter.

And, yes, I did say that there was something else that you could to do to make the job less tiring. It is as simple as this – wash up more frequently. The shorter the time you have to stand at the sink, the less tiring it is. Avoid leaving all of the washing-up until the end of the day. If you can, wash up after every meal. There is another advantage in doing this – it's good for the digestion if you stand for a while, rather than slump into a chair and compress your intestines so that they cannot function correctly.

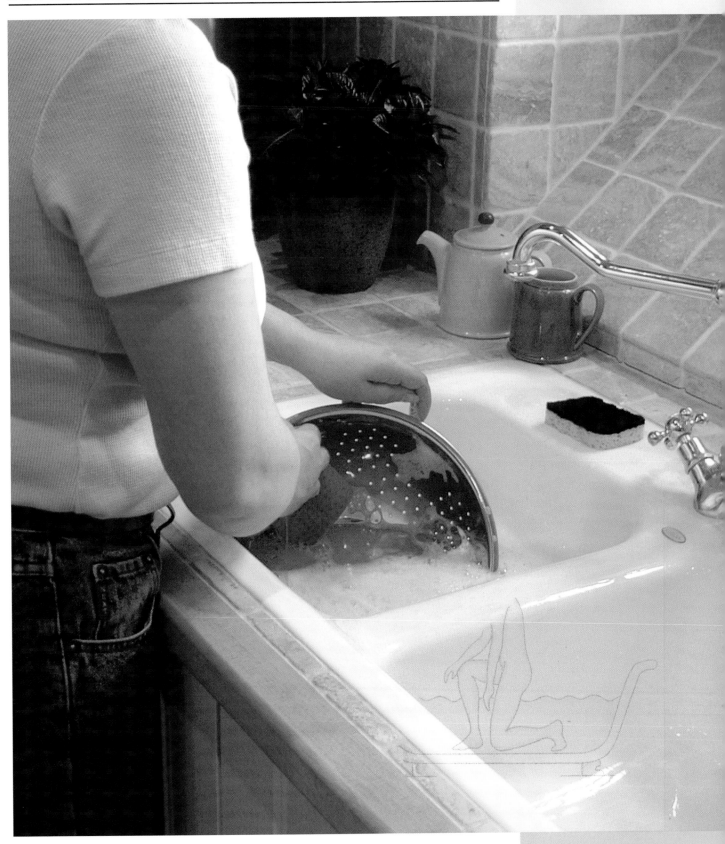

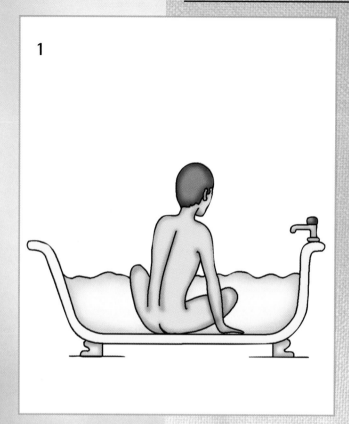

1

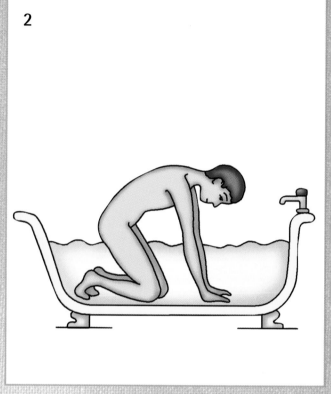

2

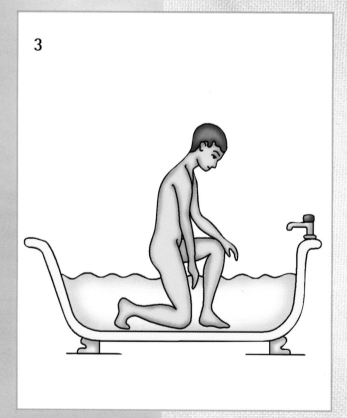

3

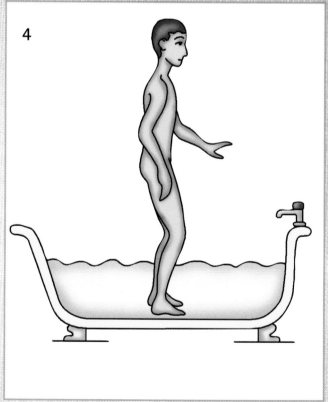

4

HAVE A BATH

After a hard day's work it's good to relax in a nice warm bath. What could be a better way to end the day? Well, having the bath is fine – the problems arise when you try to get out. Using the Alexander Technique, you can make it a lot easier and safer. Try getting out using the following steps:

1. From lying back, pull yourself up to a sitting position, holding on to the sides of the bath.

2. Then roll over so that you are on all fours, ready to crawl.

3. Bring one leg forward and up until you are kneeling on the other leg.

4. From there it is a simple move to stand up and step out of the bath.

This method allows you to get out without having to take almost your full weight on your arms – as is the usual method of getting out of the bath.

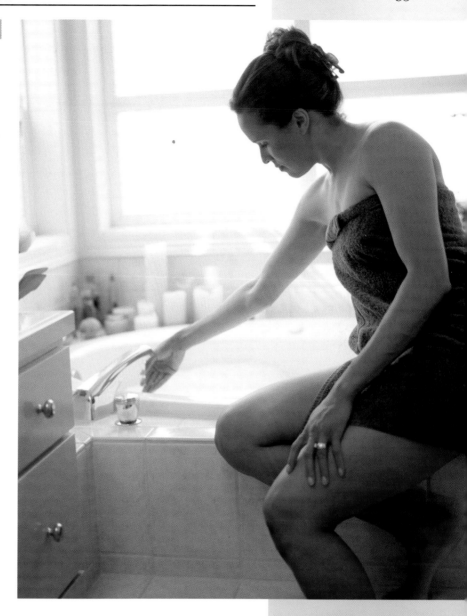

Above: after a hard day's work it's good to relax in a nice warm bath.

TO BED

And finally, it is time for bed. How can the Alexander Technique help you here? Getting into bed presents no problems. Are you going to read in bed? If so, there are two possibilities. One is to lie flat on your back with your arms up straight in the air, holding the book, which is tiring for your arms. The other is to sit up, in a normal reading posture. The difficulty here is to support your back so that you are sitting on your bottom correctly.

The tendency is to prop yourself up on one pillow and lean back against it so that your spine is curved, unsupported at its base. You are actually sitting with your weight on the bottom of your spine. This position throws your neck and head forward so that you are hunched up and cannot breathe properly.

Below: and finally, it is time for bed – again the Alexander technique can help you here.

If you like to read regularly in bed, I suggest that you buy a large foam-rubber wedge. These are available cut to size and designed specifically for this purpose. They support the full length of the spine and keep it straight and at the same time relaxed. You will find one most comfortable to use, but may find that you are so comfortable you drop off to sleep while still reading.

Now it's time to sleep. Since we move about in our sleep, it is impossible to give advice on what position to take up while asleep. The only recommendations are how to start off, get comfortable and relaxed.

Lie flat on your back. Go through the steps used when you practised lying down previously, but this time without so much of the conscious thinking:

Feel your head sinking down into your pillow.

Feel your shoulders sinking into the bed.

Feel your hips sinking into the bed.

Feel your elbows sinking into the bed.

Feel your feet sinking into the bed.

Feel your joints loosening as they relax.

Feel your spine lengthening.

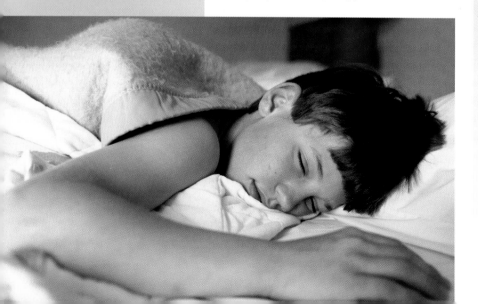

You can help with lengthening your spine by taking this in stages. After relaxing for a while, walk your heels down the bed. You'll be surprised at how far your spine stretches when you do this. After a few minutes' relaxation, do it again. Once more you will find that your spine has freed and loosened and you can walk your heels even further.

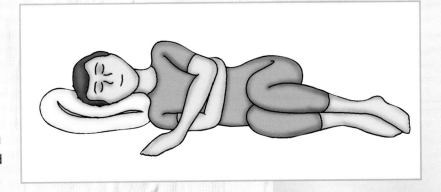

Try to remain in this position until you go to sleep. If you sleep on your back, make sure that your pillow, when pressed down, is only as thick as the books that you used when lying down on the floor. This will leave your neck free and more relaxed and your spine aligned correctly.

If you sleep on your side, you will find that you need more pillows to be comfortable – they should equal the distance from your ear to the edge of your shoulder, so that your spine remains straight, and not kinked.

Many people say that they cannot sleep on their backs or on their sides because it is uncomfortable. It is the thickness of pillow that dictates what is comfortable and what is not.

Finally, before dropping off, practise again for a few moments the whispered 'A-h-h-h-h-h'.

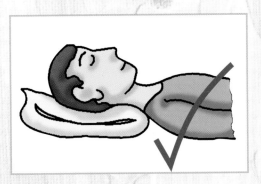

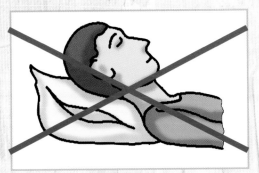

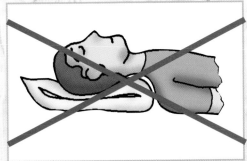

Above: if you sleep on your side, you may find that you need more pillows to be comfortable.

Left: if you sleep on your back, make sure that your pillow, when pressed down, is only as thick as the books that you used when lying down on the floor. This will leave your neck free and more relaxed and your spine aligned correctly (top left).

Alexander was wise enough to realise that many problems of posture are not caused solely through our bad habits. He looked more deeply into the relationship between mind and body and concluded that emotional stress could result in physical problems.

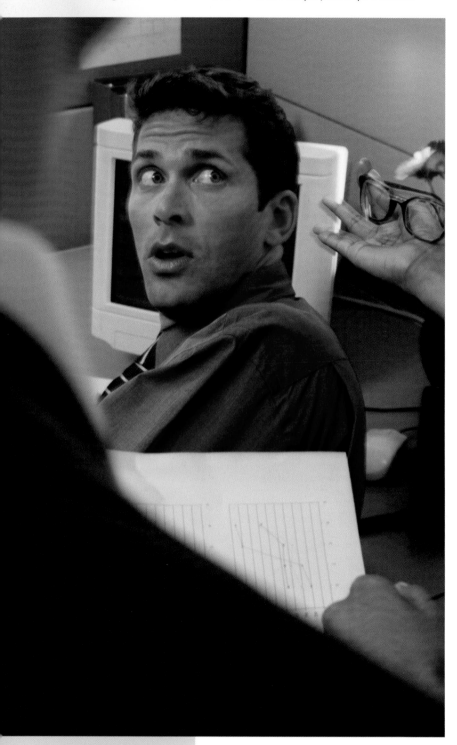

He concluded that the greatest stress was caused through fear. This emotion brings out the 'flight or fight' response that causes immediate changes to our body.

Our greatest fears are founded in threatening situations that will evoke the following involuntary physical responses:

1. Adrenalin is released into the bloodstream.

2. The hormone cortisol is released into the bloodstream.

3. The pulse rate is increased.

4. Blood pressure increases.

5. The bronchial tubes dilate to allow extra oxygen intake.

6. The breathing rate is increased.

7. The palms and soles of the feet perspire.

8. The pupils dilate to aid vision.

9. Reaction time is speeded up.

Even when we are not in physical danger, many of these responses are automatic. All these reactions cause our muscles to become tense – so that physically we are ready to face our adversary or flee.

We are still experiencing fears, but they have changed, and are no longer predominantly physical. Often nowadays our greatest fears concern the reactions of other people, or that our own forebodings may be realised. Let's look at some typical examples:

Will my boss find out my stupid mistake?

Will my wife find out about my affair?

Will anyone discover that I've cooked the books/robbed the till/fiddled my expenses?

Is that pain the first sign of cancer?

How can I pay off my debts?

All these fears bring on stress, with consequent muscle tension and an inability to relax.

The only answer is to become aware of your fear. Then, if you don't immediately know, find out what is causing your stress. Once you know what the problem is and where it is coming from, you can then address it.

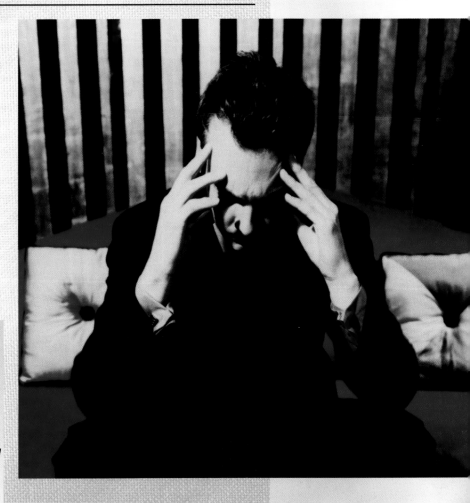

Find the solution to your fear and your stress will disappear.

Take Alexander's example. Practise his technique to relax and re-align your body.

Above: fears bring on stress, with consequent muscle tension and an inability to relax.

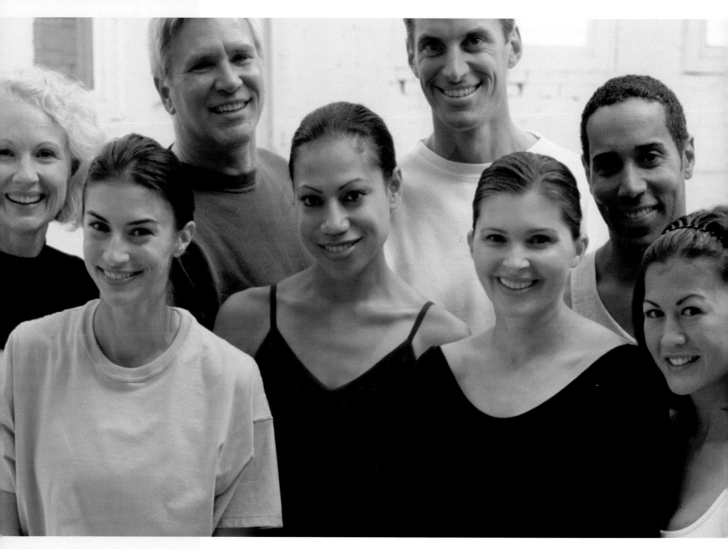

Above: the Alexander Technique is all about improving your own health and your physical and mental well-being.

The Alexander Technique is all about taking responsibility for and improving your own health and your physical and mental well-being. As you have learned, it can be used to enhance your life and bring your body back into the correct balance that is natural to it. Alexander showed us how to do this and we are all free to follow his example.

The Alexander Technique does not require you to put your hand into your pocket, as there is no equipment to purchase. Neither do you need special clothing, or have to pay to go to a gym. You can practise the technique at home. You can do it at any time, in any place. Furthermore, you can do it when you are tired, stressed or otherwise drained – something you would not want to do with any other form of physical exercise.

You may find it difficult to take on board immediately all of the exercises shown in this book – but the longest journey starts with a single step. Start with the early simple exercises and, as you become more familiar with them, move on and add to your repertoire. Gradually, as you become accustomed to the Alexander Technique you can increase your range of use until you are employing it every moment of every day. One day, with determination and practice, you will realise that the Alexander Technique has become part of your life. At this point, pause for a moment and look back to see how different you are now from how you were when you started. You will be more relaxed and easy-going, less tense, more carefree and healthier. You will look back on the way you used to hustle around, and will smile when you think how you used to be forever end-gaining and never stopping to think of the 'means whereby' you could do things in a better, easier and healthier way. Now that you are aware of it, you have regained that ease and elegance of movement that you lost when you grew out of childhood.

You have voluntarily made the conscious effort to rid yourself of your bad habits, stopped putting your body into unnatural positions and taken on a new enthusiasm for living.

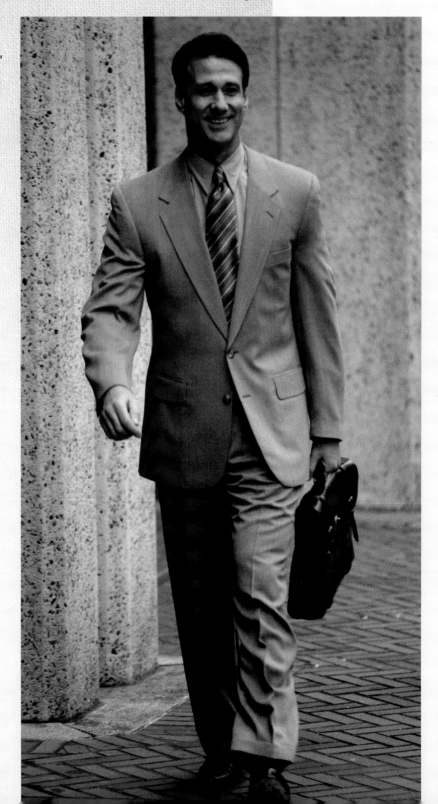

Below: one day you will realise that the Alexander Technique has become part of your life.

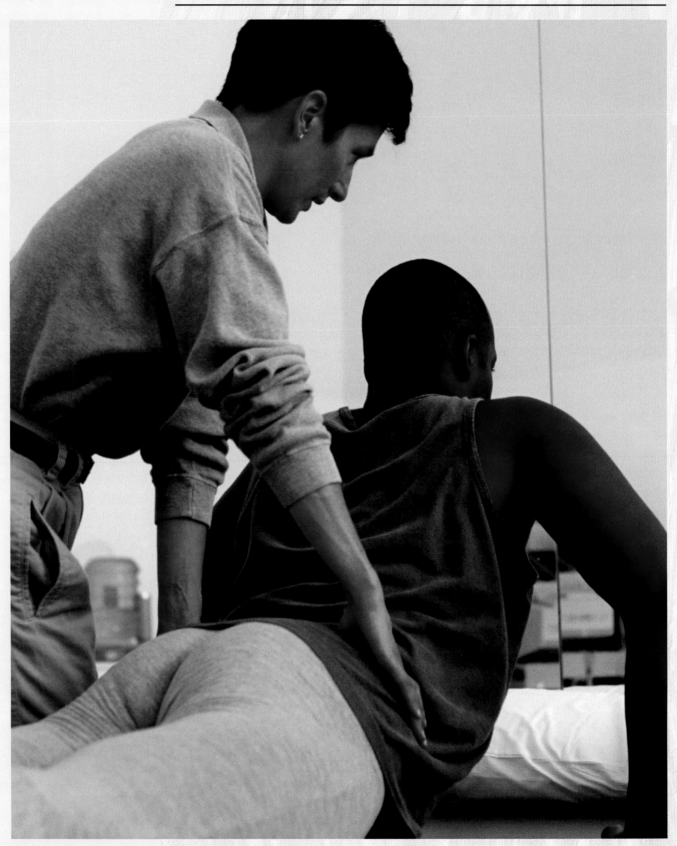

LESSONS

Although there are very few shared classes in Alexander Technique, if you need further help there are practitioners who, in the true Alexander tradition, call themselves teachers. They give lessons on a one-to-one basis.

The reason that shared classes are not held is that we are all different, each with our own weaknesses and imperfections. The teacher needs a face-to-face situation where he can correct your problems individually.

A practitioner's aim is to teach you the technique, rather than do it for you. This will then enable you to carry on practising on your own.

At your first lesson your teacher will ask you to stand, walk, sit, lie down and perhaps even read. He will then be able to assess exactly what is needed. The advantage of taking lessons with a teacher is that he will notice and correct tiny nuances of poor posture, imbalance and tension that you don't know about. You have lived with your bad habits so long that you are no longer aware of them.

If you take further lessons, you will be asked to repeat the movements mentioned earlier – walking, sitting, lying down and getting up – until the teacher is sure that you are completely aware of your body movements and have acquired a good posture. He will also make sure that you learn and understand what is meant by the various terms that Alexander used and that appear dotted throughout this book.

Becoming a fully qualified practitioner is not a quick or easy undertaking. After a rigid three-year training, recognised teachers may use the initials STAT (Society of Teachers of the Alexander Technique) after their name.

A list of practitioners can be obtained from the Society. You will find its address in the Appendix. They will also supply you with further information if you wish to become a teacher of the Alexander Technique.

Far left: a practitioner's aim is to teach you the technique, rather than do it for you.

USEFUL ADDRESSES

The Society of Teachers of the Alexander Technique (STAT) will provide you with an up-to-date list of teachers who have successfully completed an approved three-year training course.

You can also get details from them about training to become a teacher. They have a catalogue containing a large selection of books that they have for sale on the technique.

The Society of Teachers of the Alexander Technique (STAT) 20 London House 266 Fulham Road London SW10 9EL

If writing, please enclose a stamped self-addressed envelope.

Tel: 020 7351 0828 e mail: info@stat.org.uk

This is the only approved institution in the UK for training teachers of the Alexander Technique. On completion of training, teachers are included on the Society's register.

AMERICA
A.C.A.T.
129 West 67th Street
New York City
N.Y. 10023
Tel: 1 212 799 0468

AUSTRALIA
A.U.S.T.A.T.
PO Box 716
Darlinghurst
NSW 2010
Australia
Tel: (free toll from within Australia) 1800 339 571

BELGIUM
A.E.F.M.A.T.
Elizabeth Langford
4 rue des Fonds
B-1380
Lasne
Belgium
Tel: 32 2633 3059

BRAZIL
A.B.T.A.
Caixa Postal 16020
Rio de Janeiro
RJ Brazil
Tel: 55 21 239 66 18

CANADA
C.A.N.S.T.A.T.
Howard Bockner
465 Wilson Avenue
Toronto
Ontario
M3H 1TY
Canada
Tel: 1 416 631 8127

DENMARK
D.F.L.A.T.
Lis Jakobsen
Gassehaven 5
Gl. Holte
DK 2840 Holte
Denmark
Tel: 45 7025 5070

FRANCE
A.P.T.A.
Paola d'Alba
42 Terrasse de l'Iris
La Défence 2
92400
France
Tel: 33 1 4090 0623

SOUTH AFRICA
S.A.S.T.A.T.
Lynn Groll
PO Box 135
Simon's Town 7995
South Africa
Tel: 27 21 780 9412

SPAIN
A.P.T.A.E.
Simon Fitzgibbon
Apartado 156
28080 Madrid
Spain
Tel: 34 91 532 01 05

SWITZERLAND
S.V.L.A.T.
Postfach
CH 8032 Zürich
Switzerland
Tel: 41 201 03 43

There are a large number of web-sites dotted around the internet that provide interesting if not useful information about the Alexander Technique. Try keying 'Alexander technique' into any search engine and you will immediately get dozens of web-site addresses.

FURTHER READING

First and foremost must come those books written by F M Alexander himself. Most of these are still in print:

Articles and Lectures, Mouritz, 1995.

Man's Supreme Inheritance, Mouritz, 1996.

Constructive Conscious Control of the Individual, STAT Books, 1997.

The Use of the Self, Gollancz, 1996.

The Universal Constant in Living, Mouritz, 2000.

Other useful books:

Barlow, W
The Alexander Principle, Gollancz, 1973.

Craze, R
Alexander Technique, Hodder and Stoughton, 1996 & 2000.

Drake, J
The Alexander Technique in Everyday Life, Thorsons, 1996.

Gray, J
Your Guide to the Alexander Technique, Gollancz, 1998.

Leibowitcz, J, & Connington, B
The Alexander Technique, Harper and Row, 1990.

Macdonald, G
Alexander Technique, Hodder and Stoughton, 1994

Macdonald, G
The Complete Illustrated Guide to Alexander Technique, Element Books, 1998.

Macdonald, R, and Ness, C
The Secrets of Alexander Technique, Dorling Kindersley, 2001.

INDEX

A

adrenalin 86
airways 18, 44–45
Alexander technique
  'applied inhibition'49
  bathing 83
  computers 58–60
  'conscious projections'
    31–34
  digging 71
  driving 64–66
  end-gaining 75, 89
  exercise 74
  gardening 69–73
  getting out of bed
    50–51
  going to bed 84
  history of 10–12
  housework 76–80
  ironing 79
  keyboard 58–60
  lessons 91
  lifting 53–54
  monkey stance61–62
  'patterns of misuese'14
  position of
    mechanical advantage
    61–62
  practitioners 91–92
  primary control16–46
  principles of 14–15
  reading 56
  riding a bicycle67–68
  sewing 78
  sweeping up 73
  teachers 91–92
  'the means whereby'
    47, 49, 89
  training 91
  washing up 80
  weeding 72–73
  wheelbarrows 70
  'whispered Ah'44–46,
    85
  writing 57–58
Alexander Technique,
Society of Teachers
  of the 91–92

Alexander, Frederick
Matthias 9, 10–12, 43,
    46, 61, 86
alignment 11, 14, 16,
    61–62, 87
America 12
ankles 36, 53–54, 62,
    68, 70, 72
'applied inhibition' 49
arms37, 53, 60, 61–62,
    65, 67
Australia 10, 12

B

back 7–8, 16, 31, 44,
  47, 61, 74, 76, 77, 79
balance 37, 61–62, 88,
    91
bathing 83
bed 50–51, 84
bending 61–62, 69, 70,
    71
bike riding 67–68
blood pressure 9, 86
breaks, taking60, 64, 72
breathing 15, 18, 19,
  22, 24, 26, 28, 30,
    44–46, 74
bronchial tubes 86
burn-out 74
buttocks 62

C

car driving 64–66
chairs 39, 42, 43, 56,
  57, 59, 78, 79
children 7, 12, 15, 89
circulation 15, 42
clothing 18, 61, 88
coccyx 42
computers 6, 58–60
'conscious projections'
    31–34
copy-typing 59
cortisol 86
cycing 67–68

D

Dart, Raymond 16
depression 9

desktop 57, 60
diaphragm 19
digestion 7, 15, 80
digging 71
driving 6, 7, 64–66

E

elbows 24, 57, 68, 79,
    84
emotional stress 86
end-gaining 75, 89
energy 74
exercise 74, 88

F

fear 86–87
feet 24, 32, 34, 84, 86
fingers 57–60
focus 75
frozen shoulder 8

G

gardening 8, 69–73
getting up from lying
    27–28
Goldenthwaite – Body
Mechanics 8

H

habit14–15, 49, 78, 86,
89
handlebars 68
hands57–60, 61–62, 65
head16, 24, 31, 44–45,
47, 59, 61, 65, 74, 80, 84
heels 36–37, 61, 85
hernia 53
hips 24, 36–37, 40, 42,
    84
housework 76–80

I

internal organs 19
intestines 80
ironing 79

J

jaw 46
joints 7, 24, 84

K

keyboard   6, 7, 58–60
kneeling   72
knees36, 40, 53–54, 67,
          72–73, 80

L

legs   30, 34, 51, 64,
       67–68, 72–73, 83
lessons   91
lifting   8, 49, 69, 70
lungs   7, 19, 24, 45
lying down   17–26, 27,
          83, 84, 91

M

mechanical advantage,
position of   61–62
mental outlook   15
mental relaxation   76
mind-body connection
          9, 15, 76, 86
mountain bikes   68
mouth   45–46
mowing the lawn   73
muscle tension   15, 87
muscles   7, 32, 44, 47,
       51, 54, 60, 61, 67, 69

N

National Health Service
(NHS)   8
neck11, 16, 31, 44–45,
       47, 59, 61, 65–66, 74,
                    76, 80

O

oxygen   22, 74, 86

P

pain barrier   74
'patterns of misuse' 14
pelvis21, 42, 43, 56, 62
pillows   84–85
poise   37
posture 6, 7–9, 11–12,
       14–15, 56, 57, 62, 86,
                      91
practitioners   91–92
primary control   16–46

public speaking   45
pulse   86
pupils   86

R

reaction   86–87
reading   56, 91
recreation   74
regional pain syndrome
                       8
relaxation9, 11, 22, 24,
            26, 66, 87
repetitive strain injury
  (RSI)   7–8
rest   9
rhythmic movement37,
                      77
running   75
rupture   54

S

saddles   68
screen   59–60
seat belt   66
seat position   65
sewing   78
shopping   54
shoulders24, 34, 53–54,
       57–59, 62, 80, 84–85
sitting   7–8, 15, 47, 78,
                  83, 91
sitting down   39–42
sleep 9, 17, 24, 84–85
slouching   6, 7, 43, 56
slumping 7, 30, 66, 80
sound   22, 45–46
spine 7, 11, 21, 24, 43,
          62, 84–85
sports   74
standing7–8, 15, 27–28,
       30–31, 34, 44, 47,
          61–62, 91
standing up   43, 72, 83
steering wheel   64–66
stomach   7
stress68, 76, 79, 86–87
sweeping up   73
swimming   75

T

teachers   91–92
tennis elbow   8
tenosynovitis   8
tension 30, 34, 44, 47,
       56, 65, 68, 80, 91
thighs   42, 62
thinking   22, 74
toes   32, 36
tongue   45
touch-typing   60

V

vacuum cleaner   77
vision   56, 59, 86
vocal chords   46
voice   10–12, 44–46

W

walking   35–37, 91
washing up   80
weeding   72–73
weight distribution 32,
       36, 40, 42, 53–54, 66,
          71, 72, 77, 79
well-being   15, 76, 88
wheelbarrow   70
'whispered Ah'   44–46,
                      85
working surfaces57, 60,
                  79–80
wrists   60, 65
writers' cramp   8, 58
writing   57–58

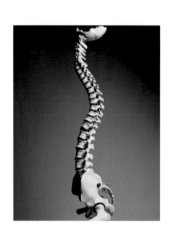